Evaluation Beyond Exams
in Nursing Education

Robin Donohoe Dennison, DNP, APRN, CCNS, CEN, CNE, is dean, Doctor of Nursing Practice Program for Chamberlain College of Nursing, and president, Robin Dennison Presents, Inc. She is an experienced clinician in the critical care arena and has taught for over 35 years. She has published widely and delivered numerous local, national, and international presentations (American Association of Colleges of Nursing, American Association of Critical-Care Nurses [AACN], Society of CNS Education, Sigma Theta Tau International [STTI], and National Association of Clinical Nurse Specialists [NACNS]). Dr. Dennison has been actively involved with her company, running certification review workshops for PCCN and CCRN certification. Three of her *Pass CCRN®!* books have received the *American Journal of Nursing* Book of the Year awards. She has also contributed to industry journals, including the *Journal of Continuing Education in Nursing, American Nurse Today, American Journal of Nursing,* and *Nursing Clinics of North America,* and recently guest edited an issue of *Nursing Clinics of North America* on the future of advanced practice nursing. Dr. Dennison is actively involved in a multitude of professional organizations, including STTI, Society of CNS Education (vice president and founding member), NACNS, National League for Nursing, American Nurses Association, and AACN.

John Rosselli, MS, RN, FNP-BC, CNE, is the director (interim) of the Nurse Educator Program and instructor at Georgetown University, Washington, DC. He is currently a PhD candidate at the University of Wisconsin–Milwaukee. Since 2007, Mr. Rosselli has taught both undergraduate and graduate levels at Georgetown University. His teaching course load has included Philosophical and Theoretical Foundations of Nursing, Technology in Teaching, undergraduate Health Assessment and Clinical Nurse Competencies, Advanced Health Assessment, Advanced Concepts of Pharmacology, and Professional Aspects of the Advanced Practice Nurse. He currently serves on the Certified Nurse Educator Test Development Committee at the National League for Nursing.

Anita Dempsey, PhD, MSN, APRN, PMHCNS-BC, is assistant professor at Wright State University in Dayton, Ohio, and director of the Psychiatric/Mental Health Nurse Practitioner Program developed through a joint appointment with the Dayton VA Medical Center. She is an experienced clinician, has taught nursing since 1986, has published six peer-reviewed articles, and has been an invited speaker at national and international conferences. Dr. Dempsey's topics focus on the scholarship of teaching and learning, professional issues, mental health issues (including the relationship between attention deficit hyperactivity disorder and obesity), safety, mental health simulation, and mental health services in disasters. She is active in the International Society of Psychiatric Nurses and currently chairs the annual conference planning committee.

Evaluation Beyond Exams in Nursing Education

Designing Assignments and Evaluating With Rubrics

Robin Donohoe Dennison, DNP, APRN, CCNS, CEN, CNE
John Rosselli, MS, RN, FNP-BC, CNE
Anita Dempsey, PhD, MSN, APRN, PMHCNS-BC

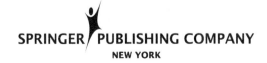
SPRINGER PUBLISHING COMPANY
NEW YORK

Springer Publishing Company, LLC
11 West 42nd Street
New York, NY 10036
www.springerpub.com

Acquisitions Editor: Margaret Zuccarini
Composition: S4Carlisle Publishing Services

ISBN: 978-0-8261-2708-2
e-book ISBN: 978-0-8261-2709-9
Rubrics ISBN: 978-0-8261-2904-8

Rubrics are available from www.springerpub.com/dennison-supplemental-materials

14 15 16 17 / 5 4 3 2 1

The author and the publisher of this Work have made every effort to use sources believed to be reliable to provide information that is accurate and compatible with the standards generally accepted at the time of publication. The author and publisher shall not be liable for any special, consequential, or exemplary damages resulting, in whole or in part, from the readers' use of, or reliance on, the information contained in this book. The publisher has no responsibility for the persistence or accuracy of URLs for external or third-party Internet websites referred to in this publication and does not guarantee that any content on such websites is, or will remain, accurate or appropriate.

Library of Congress Cataloging-in-Publication Data

Dennison, Robin, author.
 Evaluation beyond exams in nursing education : designing assignments and evaluating with rubrics / Robin Donohoe Dennison, John Rosselli, Anita Dempsey.
      p. ; cm.
 Includes bibliographical references and index.
 ISBN 978-0-8261-2708-2—ISBN 0-8261-2708-8—ISBN 978-0-8261-2709-9 (e-book)
 I. Rosselli, John (John Gary), 1970- author. II. Dempsey, Anita, author. III. Title.
 [DNLM: 1. Education, Nursing—methods. 2. Educational Measurement. 3. Educational Status. 4. Teaching—methods. WY 18]
 RT73
 610.73071'1—dc23
                    2014014287

Special discounts on bulk quantities of our books are available to corporations, professional associations, pharmaceutical companies, health care organizations, and other qualifying groups. If you are interested in a custom book, including chapters from more than one of our titles, we can provide that service as well.

For details, please contact:
Special Sales Department, Springer Publishing Company, LLC
11 West 42nd Street, 15th Floor, New York, NY 10036-8002
Phone: 877-687-7476 or 212-431-4370; Fax: 212-941-7842
E-mail: sales@springerpub.com

Printed in the United States of America by Courier.

To all my previous colleagues and students who taught me what I am now able to share in this book.

—Robin Donohoe Dennison

To my family and friends, without whom I would not have been able to participate in this project!

—John Rosselli

To my family for their enduring support.

—Anita Dempsey

CONTENTS

PREFACE

As nurse educators, we understand the goal of any nursing program is to graduate competent nurses who are prepared to provide safe care and participate fully within a complex health care system. Our success as educators depends on it. Thus the need for assessment and evaluation of achievement of student-learning objectives is vital. Undoubtedly, the primary method of student evaluation is through the administration of examinations. We spend many hours preparing examinations that are reliable and valid, often to varying degrees of success. As a result, we often evaluate our students' ability to practice effectively based on how successful they are in achieving a passing grade on multiple-choice exams.

As instructors, we all know the ability of students to pass an examination does not necessarily guarantee their effectiveness in the application of knowledge in practice. We also know that examinations are not an effective means to evaluate all learning objectives. There are other ways of evaluating student learning that can be as, if not more, effective in many situations as examinations. However, alternative evaluation strategies can be time-consuming to create and challenging to grade in a timely and consistent manner. Many educators stop just shy of providing a systematic method for assessment, evaluation, and grading.

Our initial goal was to create a book of scoring rubrics specific to common and frequently used assignments that could be easily individualized by the educator for use in assessment and evaluation of achievement of student-learning objectives in his or her course. As we embarked on this project, and considered the prospective reader may be new to nursing education, we thought it may be helpful to provide an overview of how evaluation and rubrics fit within the larger nursing education teaching–learning process as more than just a final destination or afterthought. Rubrics should be created with intent, taking into account the student-learning objectives and the teaching–learning process. With this in mind, Part I of this book provides a quick overview of the teaching–learning processes that drive and impact student assessment and evaluation. Part II provides descriptions, uses, and supporting evidence for commonly used assignments. Part II also includes detailed modifiable grading rubric templates for each assignment presented. **These modifiable grading rubric templates, found in Chapters 6 to 14, as well as some forms and tables in Chapters 3 and 4, are available to the reader at www .springerpub.com/dennison-supplemental-materials.**

This book provides practical support for the design of meaningful assignments and provides a process for effective and objective assessment, evaluation, and grading. We hope that the assignment descriptions and rubric templates will enable you to more quickly design assignments relevant to your course objectives, and to more confidently use evaluation strategies beyond examination.

Robin Donohoe Dennison
John Rosselli
Anita Dempsey

Evaluation Beyond
Examinations

How much effort do you, as a nursing educator, put into the design and development of methods for the evaluation of student learning and achievement? While it is a fundamental expectation, we often fail to address evaluation methods until after we develop the course. However, evaluation is a fundamental aspect of every course and drives the course development. While designing courses, we must consider what we want the student to learn, the scope of the learning that is needed, and how we can reasonably expect to know that the student has indeed learned what was needed. From the beginning, we need to consider what we expect the student to do or achieve as a result of completing the course and how we will know that the student is successfully progressing in that direction. Evaluation methods cannot merely be an afterthought used generically out of habit or familiarity. Rather, meaningful evaluation methods must be a forethought considered as we develop the course and integrated as learning experiences to facilitate student learning as well as to measure student achievement. Because student learning is the goal for every course, the evaluation of student learning is the ultimate measure of our success as educators. Therefore, we must design and develop evaluation methods with a clear understanding of the objectives of the course and the terminal outcomes of the program before we develop the course.

When reviewing books and articles on evaluation of student learning, the preponderance of information is about writing quality examination items with appropriate difficulty and discrimination. While examinations are certainly important, especially in prelicensure and advanced practice programs, they are not the only method of evaluation of student learning. There are a variety of teaching strategies to facilitate learning across the spectrum of cognitive, affective, and psychomotor domains. Further, within those learning domains, there is a range of levels (i.e., hierarchies) from simple (i.e., low level) to complex (i.e., high level) that can also be specifically addressed. Therefore, a wide variety of teaching/learning strategies are employed to facilitate learning across this learning matrix. Similarly, evaluation methods must be designed to reflect evaluation of learning in the appropriate domain and at the appropriate level. While examinations may be well-suited to measure achievement of knowledge, comprehension, and application of information, they are not well-suited to measure higher-level learning in the cognitive domain such as analysis, synthesis, and evaluation. In addition, adult learning theory explains that adults learn and may best demonstrate that learning in a variety of ways. Limiting evaluation to examinations may therefore limit the success of an adult in which other examination methods may be more appropriate.

The process for the evaluation of student learning is illustrated in Figure 1.1 and described in Part I of this book. Part II provides detailed discussion of a variety of assignments that educators can use for student evaluation. A modifiable analytic scoring rubric is included for each assignment type to promote the ability of the educator to easily integrate a variety of assignments into the course evaluation plan.

Evaluation of student learning starts with the process of determining student-learning outcomes at the curriculum level, which provides the framework for establishing student-learning objectives at the course level. Student-learning objectives refer to the knowledge, skills, attitudes, and values you expect your students to achieve by the conclusion of your course (Bastable, 2014; Billings & Halstead, 2011). Chapter 2 provides the tools necessary to create

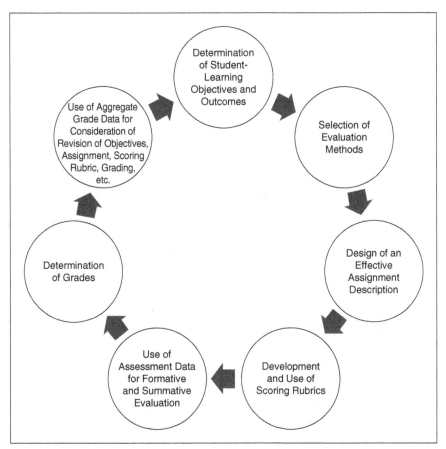

FIGURE 1.1   The evaluation process with incorporation of assignments.

effective student-learning objectives, including the use of Bloom's taxonomy. These objectives will provide the framework for creating course evaluation methods that measure your students' achievements toward those student-learning objectives.

Establishing an evaluation plan and designing assignments clearly linked to the course's student-learning objectives is the focus of Chapter 3. It is crucially important to match evaluation methods to the objectives, and each evaluation method should be matched to one or more of the course's student-learning objectives. Also in Chapter 3, methods for writing an assignment description that aid the student in understanding the reason for the assignment and promotes student success are discussed.

Rather than writing examination items, use of assignments for evaluation of student learning involves developing scoring rubrics to improve objectivity and consistency in scoring assignments. Chapter 4 differentiates types of rubrics and provides a process for developing rubrics that can be used to clarify assignment expectations and to effectively score student work products for formative or summative evaluation purposes. A step-by-step approach to developing an analytic scoring rubric is provided.

Concepts fundamental to assessment and evaluation of student achievement of learning objectives are discussed in Chapter 5. Assessment and evaluation methods directly linked to your course's student-learning objectives are essential for formative and summative evaluation. Students demonstrate achievement of the student-learning objectives via a variety of methods that extend beyond examinations when provided the opportunity. Valid methods to reliably score assignments are essential to measuring the achievement of student-learning objectives. There is much confusion about the difference between assessment and evaluation. This is clarified in Chapter 5, along with the difference between formative and summative evaluation. The use of assessment data for summative evaluation and grading is included, as well as ethical considerations of grading.

The intent of this book is to encourage you, the educator, to consider using *assignments* as an alternative or supplement to examination methods of evaluation and to do so effectively. This book provides a basic understanding of processes involved in evaluation that can be used as a quick reference. Because some educators view student evaluation through assignments as highly subjective, this book provides guidelines for designing comprehensive and well-written assignment descriptions to increase assignment clarity and provide more objective evaluation criteria. Well-written rubrics improve the chances of success for students. At the end of each chapter describing an assignment type in Part II, the authors provide a modifiable scoring rubric that can be easily adapted to reflect and to improve the objectivity of scoring those assignments.

The following terms will be used liberally in this book; these definitions are included to clarify the meaning of these crucial and sometimes confusing terms.

Analytic rubric: A rubric with at least two individual criteria that are scored separately and where the criteria are described incrementally in respect to quality (Billings & Halstead, 2011).

Assessment: The process of obtaining evidence for a specific purpose; in education, this is to obtain evidence of student knowledge and performance to understand and improve student learning.

Assignment: A task that produces a tangible work product that is used to evaluate student learning.

Evaluation: The process of assigning a value to student products such as tests, papers, presentations, and so forth, for the purposes of determining the level at which the student understands the course content. Evaluation may be formative or summative.

Formative evaluation: The collection of student-specific evidence related to the student's progress toward achievement of one or more learning objectives learning objectives and effectiveness of teaching/learning strategies. This type of evaluation takes place prior to when the student is expected to have achieved each learning objective and no grade is assigned.

Grading: The process of quantifying assessment data and assigning a value, usually A through F or a percentage, that represents the overall quality of the work. Grading is the result of summative evaluation.

Holistic rubric: A rubric that groups together several criteria and provides only a single score based on an overall impression of a student's performance on a task.

Scoring: The act of awarding points that will be converted to a percentage of possible points and then to a grade according to the established grading scale and grading policies.

Student-learning objectives: The knowledge, skills, attitudes, and values you expect your students to achieve by the conclusion of your course.

Student-learning outcomes: The expected qualities, characteristics, and/or competencies that the learner should know or be able to do by the end of a program of study.

Summative evaluation: The evaluation of student achievement of the course's learning objectives to provide feedback and assign a grade. Summative evaluation occurs at the completion of instruction so may occur with completion of a module or modules, at midterm, or at final exam.

Determination of Student-Learning Objectives and Outcomes

The goal or desired outcome of any nursing program is to graduate competent nurses who are prepared to provide safe care and participate fully in an ever-changing and increasingly complex health care system. A faculty committed to practice excellence and a curriculum that is focused on student-learning outcomes and objectives support this goal. Successful nursing graduates will leave their institutions of higher learning instilled with the knowledge, skills, attitudes, and values required of those entering the nursing profession.

This chapter discusses the effective development of student-learning outcomes and objectives related to the teaching–learning process and the design phase of curriculum development, with an emphasis on the differences between student-learning outcomes and objectives. The chapter also discusses the classification of outcomes and objectives using Bloom's taxonomy, and their effective development and implementation across all levels of the teaching–learning-assessment process, especially the student evaluation process.

By the end of this chapter, you will learn how to:

- Distinguish learning outcomes from learning objectives
- Classify learning objectives by domain and level using Bloom's taxonomy
- Develop effective learning outcomes and learning objectives

STUDENT-LEARNING OUTCOMES

In the design phase of nursing curriculum development, faculty must develop broadly stated goals that describe the nursing student's expected qualities and characteristics (Billings & Halstead, 2011). This includes what the student should know or be able to do by the end of his or her program of study (The Learning Management Corporation, n.d.), such as an undergraduate nursing program. These student-learning outcomes are student centered and are also called also called program terminal objectives, program outcomes, or program goals.

Educators create programmatic student-learning outcomes to reflect the expectations of the nursing profession, and meet the minimum standards of clinical practice (Billings & Halstead, 2011). Student-learning outcomes are not meant to describe the highly specific short-term objectives or skills-related competencies students will achieve by the end of a teaching session or specific course. Rather, these statements represent long-term programmatic goals that may take months, or even years, for students to achieve. Because student-learning outcomes reflect an accumulation of knowledge over time, they are difficult to observe and measure through discrete course assignments or other methods of student evaluation.

The example in Box 2.1 illustrates some end-of-program BSN student-learning outcomes developed for the University of Maryland School of Nursing. Note how these student-learning outcomes consist of broadly written generalized statements. This is intentional. For each of these student-learning outcomes, ask yourself if the outcome can be easily and fully measured through a single course assignment, examination, or scholarly paper. The answer should be no.

BOX 2.1

BSN Program Outcomes for the University of Maryland School of Nursing

By the end of the program, the student will be able to:

- Adhere to ethical, legal, and regulatory mandates and professional standards for nursing practice
- Use evidence-based knowledge from nursing and related disciplines to shape practice
- Provide nursing care that reflects sensitivity to physical, social, cultural, spiritual, and environmental diversity of persons
- Accept personal accountability for life-long learning, professional growth, and commitment to the advancement of the profession

Adapted from University of Maryland School of Nursing (2013).

Clinical Pearl

Write your program's student-learning outcomes to represent broad, long-term programmatic goals that take months, or even years, for students to achieve. Are these outcomes easily and fully measured through a single course assignment, an examination, or scholarly paper? The answer should be no.

The creation of student-learning outcomes is influenced by myriad factors including:

- Organizing frameworks used to influence and support the program's curriculum such as current American Association of Colleges of Nursing (AACN) baccalaureate, master's, and

DNP *Essentials* documents; national exam blueprints for the National Council Licensing Examination (NCLEX); National Council of State Boards of Nursing (NCSB); and the Institute of Medicine (IOM)

- Accrediting bodies including the Commission on Collegiate Nursing Education (CCNE) and the Accreditation Commission for Education in Nursing (ANEC)

- Credentialing organizations (e.g., American Nurses Credentialing Corporation [ANCC])

- Parent institution's and nursing department's philosophy, mission, vision, and values

- Needs of the community (local and global)

- Needs of the learner (i.e., what does the learner need to know by the end of this program?)

- What the learner should know to meet the expectations of the current and future nursing profession, and meet the minimum standards of clinical practice

STUDENT-LEARNING OBJECTIVES

Because student-learning outcomes are broad statements describing long-term goals of student achievement, each learning outcome must be operationalized and defined by more specific, short-term, measurable student-learning objectives (Bastable, 2014). Student-learning objectives, sometimes called learning objectives, identify the specific knowledge, skills, attitudes, and values, sometimes called competencies, that students must possess in order to ultimately attain the broader end-of-program learning outcomes (Bastable, 2014; Billings & Halstead, 2011) already described. Learning objectives are student focused, and do not represent the specific objectives of the educator (e.g., teaching strategies and teaching resources). They reflect the expected learning that comes as a "result of instruction, not the process or means of instruction itself" (Bastable, 2014, p. 426).

Clinical Pearl

Student-learning objectives identify the specific knowledge, skills, attitudes, and values students must possess in order to ultimately attain the broader end-of-program learning outcomes, graduate, and become successful members of the nursing profession. Student-learning objectives are measurable through assessment/evaluation measures such as examinations, course assignments, and observations in the clinical setting.

Student-Learning Objectives at All Levels of the Curriculum

Student-learning objectives are utilized across multiple levels of the curriculum to identify the specific knowledge, skills, attitudes, and values, sometimes called competencies, that students must possess at a predetermined time within the student's program of study. These times include at the end of a teaching session or series of sessions, at the end of a course, or after a particular level of instruction (e.g., sophomore year). At these particular times, student-learning objectives may refer to the competencies students are expected to achieve at the conclusion of a:

- Teaching session or a series of sessions (Bastable, 2014), often called *unit* objectives
- Course, called *course* objectives
- Particular *level* of instruction, such as the end of the freshman, sophomore, junior, or senior year, called level objectives

In all cases, the instructor should create student-learning objectives that are measurable. Table 2.1 provides examples of behavioral learning objectives at each level of the teaching–learning assessment process.

TABLE 2.1   Examples of Unit, Course, and Level Objectives

Type of Objectives	Example Objectives
	By the end of unit/course/level, the student will be able to:
Unit	• Define the nursing process • Describe the five steps of the nursing process
Course	• Develop an individual patient's plan of care using the nursing process
Level	• Apply the nursing process in the provision of care for a variety of complex patients

Clinical Pearl

Be aware, and tolerant, of how others refer to the terms student-learning outcomes and objectives. These terms are often interchanged. Outcomes may sometimes be referred to as program goals or terminal objectives, and objectives may be referred to as competencies or outcomes.

WRITING EFFECTIVE STUDENT-LEARNING OBJECTIVES

Well-written student-learning objectives provide students with a clear set of learning expectations. Through these learning objectives, "You give students clear direction for the types of performance you will accept as evidence that they have demonstrated what is expected of them" (McDonald, 2014, p. 36). There are various methods available for writing effective student-learning objectives, including specific and general formats.

Specific Student-Learning Objectives Formats

Student-learning objectives, written in a *specific* format, are measurable, narrow in scope and expectation, and closed-ended statements (Bastable, 2014). Learning objectives written in a specific format include prescriptive, clear measurements of student performance (Bastable, 2014). Consider the following specific format objective: *Following a class on diabetes, the student will be able to list at least three symptoms of type 2 diabetes.* Broken down into parts, this objective statement includes the condition or testing situation under which the student will be evaluated (i.e., following a class on diabetes). It includes who will be evaluated (i.e., the student), what the student will do or what behavior the student will perform (i.e., list symptoms), and how well the student will be able to do or master the behavior to be evaluated (i.e., at least three symptoms).

To illustrate this prescriptive format, Bastable (2014) recommends a four-part method for writing specific behavioral learning objectives (Table 2.2). Bastable based her model on Mager's (as cited in Bastable, 2014) 1997 three-part format process including performance, condition, and criterion. To this three-part process, Bastable adds a fourth element, who (p. 430). This format of writing objectives works well when developing specific, effective teaching sessions and clinical skills student-learning objectives.

TABLE 2.2   The Four-Part Method of Objective Writing

Condition (Testing Situation)	Who (Identify Learner)	Performance (Learner Behavior)	Criterion (Quality or Quantity of Mastery)
Without using a calculator	the student	will solve	five of six math problems
Using a low-fidelity model	the student	will demonstrate	the correct procedure for changing sterile dressings
Following group discussion	the patient	will list	at least two reasons for losing weight
After watching a video	the caregiver	will select	high-protein foods with 100% accuracy

Adapted from Bastable (2014).

General Student-Learning Objectives Format

By contrast, *general* student-learning objectives are not as detailed as specific student-learning objectives. General student-learning objectives often lack the condition, or testing situation, found in specific learning objectives. These statements also exclude the criterion (i.e., the quality or quantity of mastery). Consider the following example from an undergraduate health assessment course: *By the end of the course, the student will be able to perform a systematic and comprehensive health history and physical assessment on a well individual.* In this general student-learning objective, the statement identifies who will be evaluated (i.e., the student), the learned behavior to be mastered (i.e., perform), and the description of the behavior (i.e., a systematic and comprehensive health history and physical assessment on a well individual).

A general student-learning objective format is best utilized at the end of a particular teaching experience, course, or level of instruction (i.e., when or time frame). Bastable emphasizes "This format is more appropriate for stating outcomes of an academic program, when knowledge of the learner is not expected to be merely an accumulation of designated parts, but rather an integration and synthesis of broader concepts and theories over time" (Bastable, 2014, p. 430). Table 2.3 is an example of how to use this four-part method of writing general format behavioral objectives.

TABLE 2.3   Four-Part Method of Writing General Format Student-Learning Objectives

When (Time Frame)	Who (Identify Learner)	Performance (Learned Behavior)	Description of the Behavior
By the end of the course	the learner will be able to	conduct	a systematic and comprehensive health history for a well child
By the end of this module/unit/ teaching session	the student will be able to	list	the symptoms of type 2 diabetes

Adapted from Bastable (2014).

Writing Student-Learning Objectives Using Bloom's Taxonomy

Because learning objectives provide the information necessary for students to know exactly what is expected of them and when, the nurse educator must clearly articulate within the learning objective the *level* of knowledge, performance, mastery, and acquisition expected of the student, and by when. These successfully written student-learning objectives become the standards upon which you will evaluate your students.

Clinical Pearl

Successful, well-written student-learning objectives become the standards upon which you evaluate your students.

To determine the *level* of knowledge, performance, mastery, and acquisition, nurse educators often rely on Bloom's taxonomy (Bloom, Englehart, Furst, Hill, & Krathwohl, 1956), a schematic for categorizing educational learning objectives. The taxonomy successfully categorizes educational learning objectives into three interrelated domains: cognitive, affective, and psychomotor. Each domain consists of multiple levels of behavior, ordered from simple to complex, and commonly used verbs associated with those levels of behavior (Bastable, 2014; Krathwohl, 2002). Identifying the level of behavior, and the associated action verb, are critical steps in the creation of effective student-learning objectives.

Bloom's Taxonomy: The Domains

Bloom's *cognitive domain* focuses on knowledge acquisition (Billings & Halstead, 2011) and varying levels of thinking, categorized from simple to complex (Krathwohl, 2002). The cognitive domain consists of six levels of cognitive behaviors representing different levels

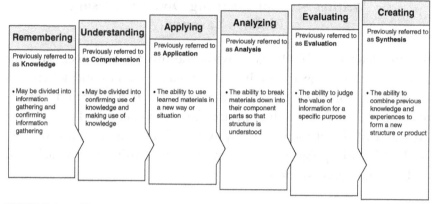

FIGURE 2.1   The cognitive domain.

Source: Adapted from Bloom, Englehart, Furst, Hill, and Krathwohl (1956).

of cognitive ability (Figure 2.1). By the end of an undergraduate nursing program, the nursing student should be performing at the highest order of cognitive skills and ability.

Clinical Pearl

"... The majority of the test items on the NCLEX are written at the application or higher levels of cognitive ability, which requires more complex thought processing" (National Council of State Boards of Nursing, 2013, p. 4). Make certain your course objectives, test items, and other methods of evaluation meet this minimum standard. Graduate student-learning objectives should also be written at the application level or higher.

The *affective domain* is often described as the "feeling" domain (Bastable, 2014). Bastable writes, "Learning in this domain involves an increasing internalization or commitment to feelings expressed as emotions, interests, beliefs, attitudes, values and appreciations" (Bastable, 2014, p. 438). The affective domain consists of five levels (Figure 2.2) of affective behavior (Krathwohl, Bloom, & Masia, 1964), which "specify the degree of a person's depth of emotional responses to tasks" (Bastable, 2014, p. 438). By the end of the program, nursing students who meet learning objectives in the affective

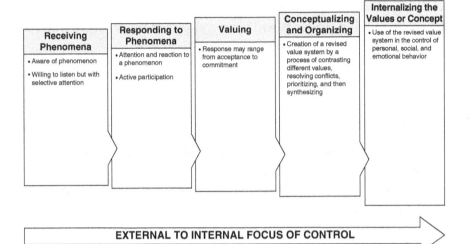

FIGURE 2.2 The affective domain.

Source: Adapted from Krathwohl, Bloom, and Masia (1964).

domain should have a better understanding of their own values, beliefs, interests, and attitudes (Bastable, 2014) through a method of self-reflection (Billings & Halstead, 2011).

The *psychomotor domain* is what nurse educators most often utilize to measure clinical practice competencies. The psychomotor domain focuses specifically on the mastery of physical skills, from simple to complex. Bloom's taxonomy categorizes these psychomotor behaviors (Figure 2.3) into seven levels ranging from perception

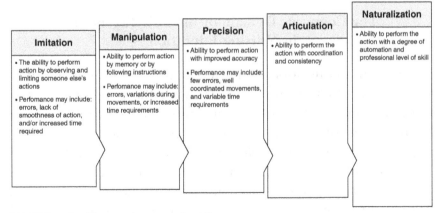

FIGURE 2.3 The psychomotor domain.

Source: Adapted from Harrow (1972).

to origination (Bloom et al., 1956). By the end of an undergraduate program, nursing students will have completed the most complex of these psychomotor behaviors.

Clinical Pearl

While there are other types of taxonomies related to educational objectives, nurse educators most often rely on Bloom's taxonomy. For more information on Bloom's taxonomy, please visit the following websites:

- Bloom's Taxonomy of Learning Domains

  www.nwlink.com/~donclark/hrd/bloom.html

- Vanderbilt University Center for Teaching

  cft.vanderbilt.edu/teaching-guides/pedagogical/blooms-taxonomy

- Bloom's Taxonomy

  www.learningandteaching.info/learning/bloomtax.htm

The Cognitive Domain of Bloom's Taxonomy in Nursing Education

Because nurse educators often evaluate through testing, and perhaps because there is unfamiliarity with the psychomotor and affective domains, they often focus on Bloom's cognitive domain when writing student-learning outcomes and objectives. Bloom's cognitive domain table (Table 2.4) will help you select the action verb (student performance) and appropriate cognitive behavior level that you expect your students to achieve by the end of a teaching session, series of teaching sessions, course, or level of

TABLE 2.4 Using Bloom's Cognitive Domain in Nursing Education

Bloom's Cognitive Level	Remembering	Understanding	Applying
Description	The ability to identify or recall information. This may involve remembering a wide range of material from specific facts to complete theories, but all that is required is the bringing to mind of the appropriate information (recalling facts only).	The ability to grasp the meaning of material. This involves translating material from one form to another (words to numbers), interpreting material (explaining or summarizing), and estimating future trends (predicting consequences or effects).	The ability to use learned material, such as facts, rules, or principles, in new and concrete situations.
Recommended verbs	**Confirming Information Gathering:** Change, match, confirm, paraphrase, express, restate, illustrate, transform **Confirming Use of Knowledge:** Extend, relate, distinguish, compare, infer, summarize, generalize, predict, defend, explain	Classify, convert, defend, discuss, distinguish, estimate, explain, express, extend, generalize, give example(s), identify, indicate, infer, interrelate, locate, paraphrase, predict, recognize, report, restate, review, rewrite, select, summarize, translate	Apply, change, choose, compute, demonstrate, dramatize, discover, employ, illustrate, interpret, manipulate, modify, operate, organize, practice, predict, prepare, produce, relate, schedule, show, sketch, solve, use, write
Evaluation by testing methods	**Confirming Information Gathering and Use of Knowledge:** Matching, true-false, and multiple-choice test items. • Who, what, when, where, how? • Define a term • Describe a process • Label a figure • Recall specific factors, concepts, principles, methods, or procedures	Fill-ins, short-answer, and most multiple-choice test items. • Retell in your own words . . . ? • What is the main idea of . . . ? To convert a knowledge-level question to a comprehension question, give a statement that includes the characteristics and ask the learner to distinguish whether it is consistent with the rule, concept, or principle.	Multiple-choice test items to assess this cognitive level require the learner to apply concepts or theories to new situations or practical settings, to solve mathematical problems, to construct graphs and charts, or to demonstrate the correct usage of a method or procedure. • How is . . . an example of . . . ? • How is . . . related to . . . ?

(continued)

TABLE 2.4 Using Bloom's Cognitive Domain in Nursing Education (continued)

Bloom's Cognitive Level	Remembering	Understanding	Applying
			• Why is . . . significant? • How could x be used to y? • How would you show, make use of, modify, demonstrate, solve, or apply x to conditions y? • Which action is indicated? Examples: Ask to identify the problem or the intervention. To convert a comprehension-level question to an application question: ask for a resultant decision or action.
Evaluation by non-testing methods	• Concept map • Case study • Reflective journaling • Minor (e.g., essays) and major paper • Presentation • Gaming (formative evaluation)	• Concept map • Case study • Reflective journaling • Minor (e.g., essays) and major paper • Presentation • Gaming (formative evaluation) • Discussion board • Presentation	• Simulation/role play • Clinical experience • Service learning • Concept map • Case study • Reflective journaling • Minor (e.g., essays) and major paper • Presentation • Gaming (formative evaluation) • Discussion board • Presentation

Bloom's Cognitive Level	Analyzing	Evaluating	Creating
Description	The ability to break down material into its component parts. This involves identifying parts, analysis of relationships between parts, and recognition of the organizational principles involved. Analyzing requires an understanding of both the content and the structural form of the material.	The ability to judge the value of material (statement, novel, poem, research report) for a given purpose.	The ability to put parts together to form a new whole. May involve the production of a unique communication (theme or speech), a plan of operations (research proposal), or a set of abstract relations (scheme for classifying information). Learning outcomes in this area stress creative behaviors, with major emphasis on the formulation of new patterns or structure.
Recommended verbs	Analyze, appraise, break down, calculate, categorize, classify, compare, contrast, criticize, deconstruct, derive, diagram, differentiate, discriminate, distinguish, examine, experiment, identify, illustrate, infer, interpret, model, outline, question, select, separate, subdivide, test	Appraise, argue, assess, attach, choose, compare, conclude, consider, contrast, criticize, critique, defend, describe, discriminate, estimate, evaluate, explain, interpret, judge, justify, predict, rate, recommend, relate, select, summarize, support, value	Arrange, assemble, categorize, collect, combine, compile, comply, compose, construct, create, design, develop, devise, explain, formulate, generate, hypothesize, invent, modify, organize, originate, plan, prepare, produce, propose, rearrange, reconstruct, relate, reorganize, revise, rewrite, set up, summarize, synthesize, tell, write

(continued)

TABLE 2.4 Using Bloom's Cognitive Domain in Nursing Education (*continued*)

Bloom's Cognitive Level	Analyzing	Evaluating	Creating
Evaluation by testing methods	Multiple-choice questions assessing this cognitive level would require the learner to integrate learning from different areas in order to view information in a new way. • What are the parts or features of . . . ? • Classify . . . according to . . . • Outline/diagram/web . . . • How does . . . compare/contrast with . . . ? • What evidence can you give (list) for . . . ? • Differentiate, compare/contrast, distinguish *x* from *y* • How does *x* affect or relate to *y*? • What piece of *x* is missing / needed? • A patient presents with these symptoms. Which of the following is the most likely diagnosis? • Scenario. Which of the following is the best action at this time?	Multiple-choice test items assessing this cognitive level would require the learner to judge the logical consistency of written material, the adequacy with which conclusions are supported by data, or the value of a work (either by internal criteria or external standards). • Do you agree . . . ? • What do you think about . . . ? • What is most important . . . ? • Prioritize . . . • How would you decide about . . . ? • What criteria would you use to assess . . . ? • Judge *x* according to given criteria. • Which option would be better/preferable to party *y*? • Scenario. Which of the following best indicates improvement/readiness to wean/etc.?	Essay questions assessing this cognitive level would require the learner to synthesize a new product utilizing multiple levels of knowledge. Not assessed with multiple-choice questions.

Bloom's Cognitive Level	Analyzing	Evaluating	Creating
Evaluation by non-testing methods	• Nursing care plan • Simulation/role play • Clinical experience • Service learning • Concept map • Case study • Reflective journaling • Minor (e.g., essays) and major paper • Presentation • Gaming (formative learning) • Discussion board	• Nursing care plan • Simulation/role-play • Clinical experience • Service learning • Concept map • Case study • Reflective journaling • Minor (e.g., essays) and major paper • Presentation • Gaming (formative learning) • Discussion board	• Nursing care plan • Service learning • Concept map • Student-created case study • Reflective journaling • Minor (e.g., essays) and major paper • Presentation • Discussion board

Adapted from multiple sources including *Task Oriented Question Construction Wheel Based on Bloom's Taxonomy* (2004); Keeley (1997); University of Oregon (2013).

instruction. In selecting appropriate cognitive-behavioral levels and action verbs, consider the following:

- **The cognitive-behavioral levels are ordered from simple to complex.** In order, the cognitive behavioral levels are remembering, understanding, applying, analyzing, evaluating, and creating. Upper-level undergraduate and all graduate nursing courses should include higher-order cognitive-behavioral objectives.

- **When writing student-learning objectives within the same level of curriculum** (e.g., teaching session objectives or course objectives), write the objective statement for the highest level of cognitive behavior desired of the student. Consider the following course objective: *Apply the nursing process in the provision of care for a variety of complex patients.* Implied in this objective is the student's mastery to recall the steps of the nursing process (remembering), and distinguish among these steps (understanding). Do not write a course objective for each of these lower-level cognitive behaviors (remembering and understanding), as their successful mastery is necessary for the student to master the stated course objective.

- **Each student-learning objective should be measureable.**

- **Each measurable student-learning objective should be achievable and realistic.** Do not evaluate students' ability to master something they have not yet learned.

- **Each student-learning objective should be measured through an appropriate evaluation process.** The measurement of student performance must be evaluated at the same cognitive behavioral level, and lower, as the stated objective. For example, if a course objective is to distinguish the symptoms associated with type 1 and type 2 diabetes (understanding), the student should not be expected to perform at a higher level of cognitive behavior analyzing lab results (analysis) via an examination question or by assignment. While lower cognitive levels of remembering or understanding can be evaluated using completion and matching questions, multiple-choice questions are appropriate for higher cognitive levels. Examples include requiring the student to select an action (i.e., applying), or to select a best, priority, or immediate action among all correct actions (i.e., analyzing), or to grade or rank findings (i.e., evaluating). Synthesizing level objectives cannot be evaluated using multiple-choice examination questions and are evaluated utilizing essay questions or one of the assignments described in the second part of this book.

- **Use only one verb per written objective.** For example, though often seen, compare and contrast should not be used. Use either compare or contrast.

Clinical Pearl

The measurement of student performance must be evaluated at the same cognitive behavioral level as the stated objective.

Clinical Pearl

As a general rule, upper-level nursing courses that have a clinical and/or lab component should include higher levels of behavior from each of Bloom's three taxonomy domains. Student-learning outcomes and objectives should include behavioral levels and verbs from each domain.

CONCLUSION

The goal of every nurse educator is to graduate competent nurses. We meet this goal by providing a curriculum that is both student and objectives focused. During the design phase of nursing curriculum development, we consider what the student should be able to know and do by the end of the nursing program. This results in the development of end-of-program student-learning outcomes that provide information to students and other stakeholders about what is expected of them and what characteristics they will possess by the end of the nursing program.

Because student-learning outcomes are intentionally broad statements describing long-term goals of student achievement, each learning outcome must be operationalized and defined by more specific, short-term, measurable student-learning objectives. These learning objectives identify the specific knowledge, skills, attitudes and values students must possess at predetermined levels within the curriculum in order to ultimately attain the broader end-of-program learning outcomes.

Effective student-learning objectives can be written in specific or general formats, depending on their purpose. Both formats should provide the student with a clear understanding of expectations related to a particular level of the curriculum. Bloom's taxonomy is a popular categorization scheme that can aid the nurse educator to write clear and effective student-learning objectives and outcomes in the three distinct yet overlapping learning domains: cognitive, psychomotor, and affective.

Design of Effective Assignments for Evaluation

After selection of student-learning objectives, you will develop a plan to evaluate the student's achievement of these objectives. Though performance on multiple-choice examinations is necessary for successful licensure and certification, a variety of evaluation methods is considered best practice for evaluation in undergraduate and graduate nursing education. The primary reason for this is that multiple-choice examinations do not readily allow evaluation of domains other than cognitive, and do not allow evaluation of higher levels of the cognitive domain. Furthermore, while critical thinking can be evaluated using well-constructed examination questions, it is also developed and evaluated through the use of alternative methods. The alternative methods of student evaluation discussed in this book may be more familiar to you as active teaching/learning strategies. When planning a course, create and select assignments that will both teach and evaluate the learning that is most important to you and the learner. Assignments designed by educators for evaluation of learning need to be worth the student's time and energy to complete, and your time and energy to grade.

By the end of this chapter, you will learn how to:

- Select alternative evaluation methods to match the domain and level of learning objectives
- Appreciate the value of a variety of methods that allow for fair evaluation of students' achievement of course learning objectives
- Develop an evaluation plan with a variety of evaluation methods that is effective in the evaluation of the course learning objectives
- Design an assignment description to increase student learning and improve a student's chance for success in producing an exemplary work product
- Describe a process to involve students in the peer evaluation of group assignments so that students earn grades according to their contribution as well as the quality of a work product

MATCHING EVALUATION TO LEARNING

As you consider the evaluation plan and assignments for your course, look first at the course student-learning objectives. In most institutions of higher learning, the curriculum committee or council of your department, school, or college of nursing develops and/or approves course student-learning objectives. The educator who is teaching the course may not be able to alter the course student-learning objectives without review and approval of the curriculum committee or council. However, the module learning objectives are generally revised at the discretion of the educator teaching the course.

As you look at the course student-learning objectives, the cognitive level of the objectives should be consistent with where the course is offered within the curriculum and the cognitive development of the student. Most course student-learning objectives at the junior or senior level of an undergraduate program and all course student-learning objectives of a graduate program should be application level or above. Senior- or junior-level undergraduate courses and graduate courses frequently include a synthesis project that demonstrates achievement of several course learning objectives. Evaluation methods with the learning domains evaluated along with examples are included as Table 3.1.

Clinical Pearl

Evaluation methods must be consistent with course learning objectives. Highest-level cognitive student-learning objectives, as well as student-learning objectives that address affective and psychomotor learning, require nonexamination evaluation methods, such as papers, presentations, reflective journaling, demonstrations, and case studies.

TABLE 3.1 Evaluation Methods With the Learning Domains Evaluated and Examples

Evaluation Method	Domain(s)			Examples
	Cognitive	Affective	Psychomotor	
Reflective journals	x	x		• Weekly reflective journal related to required readings as preparation for in-class discussion • Reflective journal related to each clinical experience
Essay	x	x		• Essay related to nursing career goals • Teaching philosophy
Scholarly paper	x	x		• Change paper describing an evidence-based practice change and using a change model • Group paper focusing on a current issue or problem in nursing

(continued)

TABLE 3.1   Evaluation Methods With the Learning Domains Evaluated and Examples (*continued*)

Evaluation Method	Domain(s)			Examples
	Cognitive	Affective	Psychomotor	
Concept maps	x	x		• Concept map showing relationship between patho-physiology and clinical presentation • Concept maps describing patient care for clinical courses
Class participation	x	x		• Contribution to discussion during class time
Discussion board	x	x		• Controversial discussions related to course content • Case studies presented for discussion
Poster	x	x		• Poster to present a published study or a synthesis of the literature on a clinical question • Poster to present a proposed change process
Case studies	x	x		• Case studies related to clinical conditions • Case studies related to workplace challenges
Presentations (individual or group)	x	x	x (if demonstration included)	• Presentation on cultural groups • Presentation on a nursing leadership issue • Video presentation of a patient history or physical examination
Simulation/ role play	x	x	x	• Simulation on patient status change or cardiac arrest • Simulation (or role play) on horizontal violence
Portfolio	X	x	x (if video included)	• Portfolio as a capstone showing evidence of achievement of program learning outcomes

DEVELOPING AN EVALUATION PLAN

In developing a student-learning evaluation plan for a course, the most important question is whether the selected methods will adequately allow for evaluation of the student's achievement of the learning objectives for the course. Each evaluation method should be an opportunity for the student to demonstrate that they achieved one or more course student-learning objectives. Consider developing a course evaluation blueprint as you would an examination blueprint (Table 3.2). Assignments also frequently contribute to experiential learning, or learning through doing. When selecting assignments for evaluation, consider that the assignment needs to be worth the student's time and energy for completion and your time for grading. Any assignment that does not link back to a course student-learning objective is "busy work."

Clinical Pearl

When selecting assignments for evaluation, consider that students should also be learning through the process of completing the assignment. If appropriate, the assignment should be enjoyable for the students and mimic an aspect of their future role. Aristotle said "for the things we have to learn before we can do them, we learn by doing them."

TABLE 3.2 Course Evaluation Blueprint Example

Objective	Exam	Participation	Presentation	Project/Paper	Other
Objective 1					
Objective 2					
Objective 3					
Objective 4					
Objective 5					
Objective 6					

When you develop your evaluation plan, consider the following points:

- **Is there a match between the cognitive level of the course learning objectives and the evaluation method for that objective?** Higher cognitive levels require methods of evaluation beyond a traditional multiple-choice examination.

- **Is there a match between the learning domain of the objective and the evaluation method for that objective?** While the affective domain can be evaluated through essay questions, other evaluation methods, such as reflective journaling or role play, are likely to be more effective. While the steps in the performance of a psychomotor skill can be evaluated through an ordering question, other evaluation methods, such as simulation or return demonstration, are likely to be more effective. These were summarized in Table 2.4.

- **Is there diversity in the selected methods of evaluation for the course?** To allow students to demonstrate their strengths, use a variety of evaluation methods (Billings & Halstead, 2011). In undergraduate courses (examinations are the predominant method of evaluation while in graduate courses), this is less likely to be true. Even in courses with evaluation predominantly by examinations, nonexamination methods in the evaluation plan are recommended to improve the chances for success for those students who do not perform well on examinations.

- **Is this going to be an individual or group assignment?** In deciding whether it will be an individual or group assignment, consider whether the assignment is usually performed by a single individual in the professional role or if the assignment is significantly complex to require the work of a group. If it is a group assignment, there needs to be some method of identifying an individual student's contribution or, more specifically, lack of contribution. A peer evaluation that can be used to seek the objective evaluation of all group members is included as Form 3.1.

Form 3.1 Peer Evaluation

Group Name: _____

Student Name: _____

Date: _____

This peer evaluation will allow you to evaluate the quality of each group member's contribution to the completion of a group assignment. Please evaluate your peers' performance and quality of work by writing in the number that best describes how well each member participated in this group activity. Please use the following rating system:

0	Frequently not present for planning sessions OR did not contribute effectively OR was counterproductive to the work of the group
1	Contributions were less than most other members of the group
2	Contributions were equal to most other members of the group
3	Contributions exceeded other members of the group

Student Names	Self	Name	Name	Name	Name
1. Participated in describing the work to be accomplished.					
2. Participated in decision making related to the group work.					
3. Contributed quality content to the group work product.					
4. Completed assignments by specified deadlines.					
5. Worked collaboratively and collegially with other group members.					
6. Exhibited professional behaviors (i.e., prompt, courteous, constructive, and respectful).					
Comments to substantiate high or low scores and identification of students' major contribution.					

Clinical Pearl

A peer evaluation method should be incorporated into group assignments to ensure that high scores are awarded to students who actually demonstrate excellence rather than reward students who do not do the work or demonstrate achievement of objectives.

- **Are the examinations and assignments manageable in terms of student workload?** Ensure that the examinations and assignments are reasonable and adequately spaced. Consider the number of credit hours for the course and the number of hours outside of class time that will be required for assigned readings, videos or webcasts, and other activities. Add the "outside of class" time required to the number of hours that would typically be required for the assignments. Take the total and divide it by the number of weeks in the course to determine the student course workload. If the student course workload exceeds 2 to 3 hours per credit hour per week, reconsider the number of examinations and/or the number and complexity of the assignments. Workloads that are excessive contribute to feelings of inadequacy and may even contribute to academic dishonesty. Also, since weaker students may require more time to complete assignments, excessive workloads could potentially set some students up to fail. Remember that given your experience and familiarity with the content being taught, you may be able to complete the assignment much quicker than a student who is doing it for the first time. How fast students "should" be able to do a particular assignment may be very different from how long it actually takes them to do it. For a new assignment, having students identify actual completion time provides valuable feedback regarding workload to be used for revision of the evaluation plan during successive offerings. If students feel overwhelmed with the workload, they must select the readings, assignment, and test preparation on which they will invest their precious time, and their priorities may not be the same as yours (Gothler, 2000).

Griffin and Novotny (2012) differentiate between minor assignments and major assignments. They describe minor assignments as being focused on something specific and likely to only take an hour or two to complete. Examples of minor assignments are an essay, journal entry, critique of a research article, response paper, brief presentation, clinical log, or debate. Major assignments include scholarly papers, presentations, or projects, and the percentage of the grade is typically commensurate with the amount of time and effort required to complete the assignment. Some types of assignments may be minor or major depending on the depth and complexity. For example, a concept map may be a minor or major assignment depending on the scope, level of detail required, and whether there is a specific or more global focus.

- **Does the percentage of overall grade of each examination and assignment match the impact of its significance in the evaluation of achievement of learning objectives?** For instance, a comprehensive final examination should be weighted more than a noncomprehensive final examination. A scholarly paper that is a synthesis of several course student-learning objectives should be weighted significantly more than an essay focused on one learning objective.

- **Are the examinations and assignments manageable in terms of faculty workload? Is it possible for you to grade and provide valuable feedback in a timely manner?** Give consideration to the educator's workload and the number of students in a class. While well-designed scoring rubrics can make grading of nonexamination methods of evaluation less time-consuming and make feedback easier to provide, assignments in general as an evaluation method are a significant time investment. If you include a scholarly paper in the evaluation plan and estimate that it will take you 1 to 2 hours to read and grade each paper and you have a class of 30 students, you are planning on investing 30 to 60 hours grading these papers for this one class. Another example is the assignment of a weekly reflective journal for a class of 150 undergraduate students, who all expect weekly feedback. This is not reasonably achievable. Also, consider whether final papers can be read and graded in time to get final grades submitted by deadline, especially for graduating seniors.

Clinical Pearl

Providing valuable feedback is more important than simply grading an assignment; while grading is important to evaluation, it is the detailed feedback that contributes to learning.

If it is appropriate to use a group assignment rather than individual assignment, the grading requirements are significantly reduced. However, the first consideration is whether the assignment is appropriate as a group assignment, as previously described.

- **Does the evaluation plan optimize chances for success?** When educators evaluate students using multiple methods of evaluation, students' chances for success improve. As a general rule, no one evaluation method should constitute more than 25% to 30% of the student's grade, since poor performance on that one examination, such as a midterm or final, or a major assignment would result in a poor grade for the course even if the student's other grades are acceptable.

- **Does the evaluation plan schedule allow for "early warning" of poor performance?** The due dates for evaluation methods need to be distributed throughout the course, with close to 50% of the evaluation plan being completed by the midterm to allow students time to improve their grade if their early performance results in a grade less than passing or is not the desired grade. Some evaluation plans are scheduled so that more than 75% of the grade is from assignments in the last 2 to 3 weeks of the course. This potentially contributes to student failure since poor performance on these late assignments does not allow the student adequate time to recover from poor performance in the course or withdraw from the course in good standing. For inclusion in a syllabus, the evaluation plan for a course should include a brief description of the evaluation method, the percentage of the grade contributed by the evaluation method, and the examination date or the due date and time for the assignment. Though some educators also include points, this can lead to students being obsessed with each and every point rather than viewing the overall evaluation plan and their overall performance. With weighting of scores, points are irrelevant and it is best to score and record everything as a percentage. Students frequently do not understand that 5 points of 25 in an assignment that is worth only 10% of the student's grade is not as significant as 5 points of 25 in an assignment that is worth 30% of the student's grade. Furthermore, students may feel compelled to argue regarding every single point, even when there may be 1,000 points total in the evaluation plan; note that in this example, 1 point is worth .001% of the student's total grade.

Clinical Pearl

Forget points! Record all grades as a percentage of the total points possible for that assignment rather than recording the number of points. Students frequently become obsessed with points even if 1 point is 1/1,000 or even 1/10,000 of their grade.

Tables 3.3 and 3.4 are examples of evaluation plans for inclusion in a syllabus for a semester course. Note that there is variety in the evaluation methods, with examinations (i.e., quizzes) accounting for only 40% of the student's grade. Also, note that no one evaluation method is worth more than 30%. Though 40% of the grade is from quizzes, each quiz is only worth 10%. Though five quizzes will be given, only the top four scores will be used in calculation of the final grade. This is helpful if a student must miss an examination or if the student does poorly on one examination. This discourages students from missing an examination unless it cannot be avoided, since the missed exam score becomes the lowest score that is excluded.

TABLE 3.3   Evaluation Plan for an Undergraduate Leadership Course

Evaluation Method	Percentage of Course Grade	Due Date
Weekly reflective journal related to assigned readings	15%	Weekly at 11:55 p.m. on Wednesday
Group project: Professional presentation on a nursing issue (group selected but professor approved)	20%	Week 10
Quizzes (5 multiple-choice quizzes with lowest score eliminated)	40% (10% x 4)	Beginning of class time in Weeks 3, 6, 9, 12, and 15
Resume and career path essay assignment	25%	Wednesday at 11:55 p.m. of finals week (Week 16)

TABLE 3.4   Evaluation Plan With Building Assignments in a Graduate Evidence-Based Practice Course

Evaluation Method	Percentage of Course Grade	Due Date
Clinical question in PICOT (i.e., problem, intervention, comparison, outcome, time) format	5%	Wednesday at 11:55 p.m. of Week 3
Key word list, search strategy, and results	10%	Wednesday at 11:55 p.m. of Week 5
Evidence table	20%	Wednesday at 11:55 p.m. of Week 10
Peer presentation on PICOT question, systematic review, and summary statement	25%	Class session of Week 15
Evaluation and feedback to peers after peer presentations	10%	Within 72 hours of peer presentations
Scholarly paper with systematic review and summary statement	30%	Wednesday at 11:55 p.m. of finals week (Week 16)

Note that these assignments build throughout the semester so that feedback from each assignment assists in learning and refinement of the final product. Since the final scholarly paper is a synthesis assignment, it is worth a significant percentage of the student's grade.

Clinical Pearl

When giving multiple quizzes or examinations, consider throwing out the lowest score; this encourages students to be present for all quizzes so that they can save their "throw out" for a quiz or examination with a poor score and avoids makeups that cause a delay in receiving grades for those students who took the quiz or examination when it was given.

WRITING AN ASSIGNMENT DESCRIPTION

When writing an assignment description, always start with the purpose of the assignment to emphasize time on task. The other crucial aspects will allow the student to be successful in completing and submitting the assignment on time, in the required format, and of the expected quality.

Purpose

When writing an assignment description, start by clearly describing the purpose of the assignment. Link the assignment to one or more of the student-learning objectives for the course to aid students in seeing the significance of the assignment. If possible, link the assignment to performance in their future role, such as registered nurse, advanced practice nurse, nurse educator, or nurse administrator.

Name and Description

The name of the assignment should clearly describe the assignment. As an example, instead of naming an assignment "Peer Presentation," name the assignment "Peer Presentation on Selected Current Nursing Issue." Clearly indicate whether the topic is assigned by the educator or selected by the student. If the topic is selected by the student, identify whether approval is required by the educator and by when. Also, if it is a group assignment, identify whether members are assigned to a group by the educator or if students are allowed to select their group members and how many members are to be in a group. Identify how and when the group membership is communicated to the educator.

> ## Clinical Pearl
>
> If you provide a complete description of the assignment, you reduce the number of questions about the assignment and increase the quality of the work product. Provide explicit directions regarding the expectations of the assignment and how it will be graded, including the scoring rubric.

Parameters

Essential elements of the assignment should be clearly identified. These are the aspects of the assignment that should be addressed in the presentation, the paper, the poster, and so on. It is helpful to refer the student to the scoring rubric, which will clearly define the expectations related to each essential element.

Format and Style

If the paper is expected to be in American Psychological Association (APA) format, that needs to be specified. The expected length in number of pages for a paper or time limit for a presentation should be identified. If you are not asking that the paper be formatted in APA, be specific about font with point size, margins, and spacing. For electronically submitted posters, you might specify that print be legible on your computer monitor at 18 inches.

> ## Clinical Pearl
>
> If you do expect an assigned paper to be in APA format, ensure that the students have received instruction and resources about APA. Remind students that following a specific style is more than just the way that references are formatted; it is also the way the paper is formatted.

Indicate whether references are required and include expectations regarding the type and number of references on the rubric. Students frequently need clarification about what you perceive as an acceptable reference. You may think that it is obvious that Wikipedia is not a professional reference, but use of this resource is so ubiquitous to students that you need to be very clear that professional references include professional journal articles, professional books, and nonbiased websites (such as those ending in .edu, .gov, or .org). If you want all or some of the references to be research reports, specify that.

Clinical Pearl

Be specific about how many and what type of references you expect. Also, indicate what types of references should not be used, such as Wikipedia or commercial (i.e., .com) websites.

You may consider providing an APA template with what is expected in each section. You may also consider providing an exemplar, such as an excellent paper from a previous student or one that you develop specifically for the purpose of serving as an exemplar. Besides getting permission from the student, one problem with using a previous student's paper is that any errors that you missed will be seen as acceptable even if they are contrary to the guidelines or the rubric description of an A paper. Also, templates and exemplars may imply that this is the only way to complete the assignment and therefore decrease creativity and innovation.

Due Dates

Specify the date and time, including time zone, the assignment is due. Consider the following aspects when setting due dates and times.

- Is there adequate time between this and other assignments or examinations?

- Is there enough time to allow students to access library resources? Assignments due early in the course that require professional references may not allow students time to procure articles through interlibrary loan if necessary.

- Does this due date conflict with other assignments or examinations in other courses, especially if all or most of the students in this course are in the another course?

There are several advantages to breaking major assignments into incremental components. It allows for formative evaluation if you are willing to review and provide helpful feedback for students to use for revision. Asking for scholarly papers in increments of outline, rough draft, and final draft reduces the risk of plagiarism and the purchase of papers. It also discourages students from procrastinating until the last minute to start work on the assignment.

Clinical Pearl

Consider asking students to screen their papers using antiplagiarism software, such as SafeAssign or TurnItIn and submit the report with their paper. Having students screen their own papers prior to submission allows them to revise their paper to avoid unintentional plagiarism.

Be specific in the assignment description regarding late submissions; will they be accepted and, if accepted, will there be a penalty? If there is a penalty of points per day for late submission, indicate whether the day count includes weekend days. Also, be specific about extensions and what constitutes as a justifiable reason for an extension and if it must be requested prior to the due date and time.

Submission Guidelines

Be very specific about how the assignment is to be submitted. Indicate whether it should be submitted in paper or electronic form.

If electronic, indicate whether it should be submitted through the assignment manager of the classroom management system or as an e-mail attachment. Also, be specific about how the file should be named. Ask students to use their last name in the file name along with an abbreviation of the assignment name. For instance, the file name for a PowerPoint presentation might be named LASTNAM-EPP.ppt or .pptx. If using e-mail and you are teaching more than one course where you have assignments being submitted electronically, it is helpful that you include the course number or name in the file name (i.e., RESEARCHLASTNAMEPP.ppt or pptx).

> ## *Clinical Pearl*
>
> Providing very specific instructions regarding how the file should be named prevents having multiple files named final paper and having to open the paper to determine who wrote the paper.

Grading

Indicate on the assignment description how the assignment will be graded. If the student will get credit for simply turning in the assignment, indicate that. Indicate if the assignment will be graded using a scoring rubric, and include the scoring rubric when you provide the assignment. Students frequently need to be reminded repeatedly to review the scoring rubric.

> ## *Clinical Pearl*
>
> Encourage students to use the scoring rubric as a checklist to ensure that all required elements are included. The scoring rubric can also be used to self-grade their paper so that they can make revisions to improve the quality of the paper prior to submission.

If a preliminary review of the paper before grading will be offered, indicate that. Establish clear guidelines regarding when the paper can be turned in for a preliminary review to avoid being overwhelmed with papers for review immediately prior to when they are actually due. Whether you can provide a preliminary review of the paper is generally dependent upon the number of students in the course and your other workload responsibilities.

Finally, be honest about your "pet peeves." We all have them so communicate yours to your students. You might even consider having a brief discussion about "common errors or omissions" with students if this is an assignment that you have used before and have seen common issues that reduce the quality of the work product.

CONCLUSION

This chapter provided a discussion regarding development of an evaluation plan along with the significance of including nonexamination forms of evaluation of learning objectives. Also included in this chapter were guidelines for writing an assignment description to improve the student's chance of success. A peer evaluation process was described for use with group assignments along with an evaluation form that may be used to obtain feedback regarding contribution of individual group members to the final work product. Descriptions of common nonexamination assignments with modifiable examples of scoring rubrics are included in Chapters 6 to 14. You can easily adapt these scoring rubrics to specific courses and assignments.

4

Development and Use of Scoring Rubrics for Objective Grading

As educators, the establishment of student-learning outcomes and methods of evaluation of the achievement of these outcomes are crucial aspects of the educational process. There are two primary reasons educators frequently choose examinations for evaluation of student-learning outcomes. The first is that grading of assignments is difficult and time-consuming. While developing a scoring rubric is a significant upfront time investment, using the rubric will reduce the time required to grade the assignment. The second reason is that educators (and students) appreciate the objectivity of a well-constructed examination. Developing scoring rubrics significantly improves the objectivity of grading nonexamination methods of evaluation. Also, sharing these rubrics with students in advance significantly improves the quality of the work by communicating clearly to the students the expectation for the assignment by incrementally showing what is required for grade or point levels. Unfortunately, research evidence is sparse regarding the use of a scoring rubric for formative or summative evaluation.

By the end of this chapter, you will learn how to:

- Describe the importance of using scoring rubrics to ensure objectivity and consistency in grading assignments
- Develop a scoring rubric for selected assignments using a step-by-step approach
- Utilize a scoring rubric to objectively score assignments
- Provide valuable feedback to students regarding achievement of student-learning objectives through assignments

WHAT IS A RUBRIC?

A rubric is a scoring tool that lays out specific expectations for an assignment. Allen and Tanner (2006) define a rubric as "a type of matrix that provides scaled levels of achievement or understanding for a set of criteria or dimensions of quality for a given type of performance, for example a paper, an oral presentation, or use of teamwork skills" (p. 197). A scoring rubric articulates criteria for different levels of student achievement for a specific assignment. Rubrics provide a criterion-based assessment process. A student's work is compared to the criteria rather than to the work of other students. The most common format for a rubric is a table or grid with the criteria in rows on the left side and the graduations of quality in columns across the top.

SCORING SHEET VERSUS A RUBRIC

To make an important distinction, what many educators call a rubric is actually not a rubric at all but rather a scoring sheet, indicating simply how many points are designated for each aspect of the assignment. Scoring sheets do not provide incremental descriptions of quality and do not reduce the time required for grading or the subjectivity of grading. They do not clearly communicate to the students the expectations of quality for each of the criteria. The educator spends an inordinate amount of time providing written feedback. Consider the example of a scoring sheet for an evidence-based practice (EBP) project paper (Box 4.1) and how limited it is in providing guidance for the student and educator, and justifying the score given.

BOX 4.1

A Scoring Sheet for an Evidence-Based Practice Project Paper

Criterion	Points Possible
APA	5
Introduction and Conclusion	5
PICOT Question	5
Significance of the Problem	10
Search Strategy and Results	10
Critical Appraisal of the Literature	15
Summary Statement	10
Clinical Recommendations	10
Planned Change Process	10
Evidence Table	15
Mechanics/Word Usage/Grammar/Punctuation	5

PICOT, problem/population, intervention, comparison, outcome, timing.

Two Primary Types of Scoring Rubrics

Holistic Rubrics

A holistic rubric groups together several criteria and provides only a single score based on an overall impression of a student's performance on a task. Characteristics of an A assignment, a B assignment, and so forth are listed but the criteria for the assignment are considered in a combined manner (Billings & Halstead, 2013). The educator then makes a judgment based on how closely the student's work product matches the score descriptions (McDonald, 2014). Holistic rubrics are more likely to be helpful to make a quick or global judgment, such as a minor assignment like a brief homework assignment. The primary advantage of holistic rubrics is that they allow quick scoring and are efficient for scoring assignments of large groups of students. Nilson (2010) attests that scoring using a holistic rubric is "relatively quick, efficient, reliable, and fair when backed by instructor experience, practice, and familiarity with the student performance range at the institution" (p. 304). Nitko and Brookhart (2011) state that holistic rubrics are preferred when there is no definitive answer or there is an overlap among the criteria. While a holistic rubric is better than a scoring sheet (Box 4.1), it does not provide students with specific feedback on their strengths and weaknesses. It may be difficult for multiple scorers to decide on one consistent overall score due to the lack of detail regarding assignment expectations. An example of a holistic rubric for an evidence-based project paper is included as Box 4.2.

BOX 4.2

A Holistic Rubric for an Evidence-Based Project Paper

Exceeds Expectations (A)	No writing and American Psychological Association (APA) errors in paper. The introduction stimulates interest and provides a preview of the paper while the conclusion provides an interesting summary. The PICOT question is stated succinctly with operational definition/descriptions of all elements of the question. The description of the problem being investigated includes current information on incidence and significance. The search strategy is thoroughly described, including search terms and the results of the literature search. The summarization of the existing evidence related to the PICOT question is complete with attention to the strength of the evidence. The narrative summary of the evidence describes the key evidence to answer the question along with a conclusive statement. There is a logical EBP recommendation and a proposed change. The choice of change model is appropriate to the recommended change. There is a description of the model and the planned change process using the model. Specific evaluation criteria are included. The evidence table includes at least 10 to 15 research articles with each study critically appraised, summarized, and accurately graded.

(continued)

Box 4.2 (*continued*)

Meets Expectations (B)	Good writing and APA style throughout the paper but a few errors. The introduction previews and the conclusion summarizes. The PICOT question is stated succinctly with brief description of all elements. There is a description of the problem being investigated. There is a description of the search strategy and results of literature search. There is a summarization of the existing evidence related to the PICOT question with attention to the strength of the evidence. There is a narrative summary of the evidence with a conclusive statement. There is a description of the EBP recommendation and proposed change. There is a description of the selected change model and planned change process using the model. Evaluation criteria are described. The evidence table includes at least 10 research articles with each study critically appraised, summarized, and accurately graded.
Nearly Meets Expectations (C)	Several writing and APA style errors in paper. Introduction does not stimulate interest or preview and conclusion does not summarize. The PICOT question is stated but there are deficiencies in element descriptions. The description of the problem investigated is brief and incomplete. The description of the search strategy and results of literature search are brief and incomplete. There is a brief and/or nonsuccinct summarization of the existing evidence related to the PICOT question. There is a fair narrative summary of the evidence with a conclusive statement. There is a description of EBP recommendation and proposed change. There is a brief description of change model and planned change process, though there is little correlation between the model and the proposed change process. Evaluation criteria are nonspecific. The evidence table includes fewer than 10 research articles and the articles are either inadequately or inaccurately critically appraised, summarized, and graded.

(*continued*)

Box 4.2 *(continued)*

Does Not Meet **Expectation (F)**	Many errors in writing and APA style throughout paper. The introduction and conclusion neither preview nor summarize. The PICOT question is stated but there are several deficiencies in element description. The description of the problem investigated is incomplete or inaccurate. The description of the search strategy and results of literature search are incomplete. There is a brief and/or inaccurate summarization of the existing evidence related to the PICOT question. There is a narrative summary of the evidence with a conclusive statement but it does not logically progress from the evidence. There is a description of the EBP recommendation and proposed change, but the change is not consistent with the evidence. There is a brief description of change model and planned change process but the change model selection is illogical and/or the actual recommended steps in the change process are not included. No evaluation criteria are included or they are not measureable. The evidence table includes fewer than 10 research articles and the articles are inadequately or inaccurately critically appraised, summarized, and graded.

Analytic Rubrics

With an analytic rubric, at least two individual criteria are scored separately and the criteria are described incrementally in respect to quality (Billings & Halstead, 2013). Criteria may include aspects such as APA, writing and grammar, or evidence of critical thinking. The primary advantages of using an analytic rubric is that it provides more detailed guidance and feedback for student performance and it promotes more consistent scoring among educators scoring the assignments. The primary disadvantage is the upfront time of developing the rubric but is certainly less time-consuming than scoring without a rubric. An example of an analytic rubric for an EBP project paper is included as Table 4.1. Note the specificity that guides the student and the educator. The remainder of this book focuses on analytical scoring rubric development.

TABLE 4.1 An Analytic Rubric for an Evidence-Based Practice Project Paper

Criterion (Points Possible)	Does Not Meet Expectations	Nearly Meets Expectations	Meets Expectations	Exceeds Expectations	Score and Comments
	≤ 3.5	3.5	4	5	
APA (5) Title page, headings, citations, reference page, font, layout, margins	Major problems with implementation of APA style in title page, headings, citations, and/or reference page. Font, layout, and/or margins do not adhere to APA format.	Missing 3–5 APA elements in title page, headings, citations, reference page, font, layout, and/or margins.	Missing 1–2 APA elements in title page, headings, citations, reference page, font, layout, and/or margins.	Fulfills APA criteria in title page, headings, citations, and/or reference page. Font, layout, and/or margins adhere to APA format.	

(continued)

TABLE 4.1 An Analytic Rubric for an Evidence-Based Practice Project Paper (*continued*)

Criterion (Points Possible)	Does Not Meet Expectations ≤ 3.5	Nearly Meets Expectations 3.5	Meets Expectations 4	Exceeds Expectations 5	Score and Comments
Introduction and conclusion (5)	Incomplete or unfocused purpose statement. There is no clear introduction of the main topic and/or the structure of the paper is missing and/or there is no summary in the conclusion.	The introduction states the purpose but does not adequately preview the structure of the paper. The conclusion is not effective in summarizing the contents of the paper.	The introduction clearly states the paper's purpose in a single sentence. The introduction states the main topic and previews the structure of the paper. The conclusion summarizes the contents of the paper.	The introduction clearly and concisely states the paper's purpose in a single sentence that is engaging and thought provoking. The introduction states the main topic and previews the structure of the paper. The conclusion effectively summarizes the contents of the paper.	

	≤ 3.5	3.5	4	5
Body: PICOT (5)	The clinical question is not in PICOT format. The elements of the question are not operationally defined or described.	The clinical question is not in PICOT format and/or the operational definitions/descriptions are poorly developed or confusing.	The PICOT question is succinctly stated but operational definitions/ descriptions of the elements of the question are poorly developed.	PICOT question is succinctly stated and includes operational definitions/ thorough descriptions of unique qualities of the population, description of the intervention being evaluated and the comparison, and the expected outcome(s) being evaluated. Timing is included if appropriate.

(continued)

TABLE 4.1 An Analytic Rubric for an Evidence-Based Practice Project Paper *(continued)*

Criterion (Points Possible)	Does Not Meet Expectations	Nearly Meets Expectations	Meets Expectations	Exceeds Expectations	Score and Comments
	≤7	8	9	10	
Body: Significance of the problem (10)	The significance of the problem is not developed through the use of current, scientific evidence. No discussion of legal, ethical, quality, or safety implications.	The significance of the problem is minimally developed with few current scientific references related to incidence and significance. Minimal or no discussion of legal, ethical, quality, or safety implications.	The significance of the problem is developed with information regarding incidence supported by current, scientific evidence. There is limited description of impact on patient/family, health care providers, institution, and health care system. Discussion of legal, ethical, quality, and safety implications is present but limited.	The significance of the problem is established through current scientific evidence regarding incidence and descriptions of the impact on patient/family, health care providers, institution, and health care system. There is a thorough discussion of legal and ethical implications as well as discussion of the impact on quality or safety.	

	≤7	8	9	10
Body: Search strategy and results (10)	The search strategy is poorly described. There is no explanation of the logic for this process. Poor description of the search results; reasons for exclusion of articles from pool of articles found not described.	The search strategy is incompletely described with omission of search words/ terms, databases used, and/or inclusion and exclusion criteria. Explanation of the logic for this process is limited. The description of the search results including number and type of articles found through each database and reasons for exclusion of articles from pool of articles found described but limited.	The search strategy is described, including search words/terms used, databases used, inclusion and exclusion criteria. Explanation of the logic for this process is brief. There is a description of the search results including number and type of articles found through each database and reasons for exclusion of articles from pool of articles found is described.	The search strategy is thoroughly described, including search words/ terms used, databases used, inclusion and exclusion criteria, and thorough explanation of the logic for this process. There is a thorough description of the search results, including number and type of articles found through each database and reasons for exclusion of articles from pool of articles found is described.

(continued)

TABLE 4.1 An Analytic Rubric for an Evidence-Based Practice Project Paper (*continued*)

Criterion (Points Possible)	Does Not Meet Expectations	Nearly Meets Expectations	Meets Expectations	Exceeds Expectations	Score and Comments
	≤ 10	11–12	13–14	15	
Body: Critical appraisal of the literature (15)	The summary lists existing evidence related to the PICOT question but does not address the quantity, quality, or consistency of the evidence.	The summary of the existing evidence related to PICOT question that addresses the number and type of studies but poor attention to the quality of the studies.	There is a summary of the existing evidence related to PICOT question that addresses the quantity, quality, and consistency of the evidence.	There is an exemplary summary of the existing evidence related to the PICOT with attention to the strength of the evidence (quality, quantity, consistency).	
	≤ 3.5	3.5	4	5	
Body: Summary statement (5)	There is a brief and/or noncohesive narrative summary of the evidence. There is no conclusive statement of the results of the systematic review or the statement does not answer the PICOT question.	The narrative summary of the evidence includes a conclusive statement of the results of the systematic review and does answer the PICOT question but the conclusive statement is not based on the highest level of evidence found.	The narrative summary of the evidence includes a conclusive statement of the results of the systematic review that answers the PICOT question with more weight given to research evidence.	The narrative summary of the evidence is succinct and includes a logical conclusive statement of the results of the systematic review. The summary statement answers the PICOT question with more weight given to research evidence.	

	≤7	8	9	10
Body: Clinical recommendations (10)	There is no clear description of a clinical recommendation or proposed practice change, or there is no linkage between the proposed practice change and the presented summary.	There is a limited description of the clinical recommendation and proposed practice change; the proposed practice change is not supported by the presented evidence summary.	This is a description of the clinical recommendation and the proposed practice change and it flows logically from the evidence presented.	This is a clear and complete description of the clinical recommendation and the proposed practice change and it flows logically from the evidence presented.

(continued)

TABLE 4.1 An Analytic Rubric for an Evidence-Based Practice Project Paper (*continued*)

Criterion (Points Possible)	Does Not Meet Expectations ≤7	Nearly Meets Expectations 8	Meets Expectations 9	Exceeds Expectations 10	Score and Comments
Body: Planned change process (10)	There is no identification of a change model. There is little or no discussion of barriers and facilitators of change or evaluation process.	The choice of change model is illogical in relation to the recommended change process. The model is not used to describe recommended steps in planned change process. There is limited discussion of the barriers and facilitators of change or the evaluation process.	The choice of change model is logical in relation to recommended change process. The change model is used to describe the recommended steps in the planned change process. There is a discussion of barriers and facilitators of change and evaluation process.	The choice of change model is logical in relation to recommended change process. The change model is used to describe the recommended steps in the planned change process and the steps are specific to the setting/institution in which the change is planned. There is an extensive discussion of barriers and facilitators of change that are specific to the change setting/institution. There is a description of criteria for evaluation and process for evaluation.	

	≤ 10	11–12	13–14	15
Appendix: Evidence table (15)	Includes fewer than 8 articles; articles are poorly evaluated and summarized and most are incorrectly graded. Grading scale is not described and/or referenced.	Includes at least 8 articles with at least 6 of them primary research articles; articles are briefly evaluated and summarized and most are correctly graded. Grading scale is described and referenced.	Includes at least 10 articles with at least 8 primary research articles; all articles are satisfactorily evaluated and summarized and correctly graded. Grading scale is described and referenced.	Includes 10–15 articles with at least 10 primary research articles; all articles are thoroughly evaluated and summarized and correctly graded. Grading scale is described and referenced.

	≤ 3.5	3.5	4	5
Mechanics/ usage (5)	Numerous and distracting errors in punctuation, capitalization, spelling, sentence structure, and word usage.	Many errors in punctuation, capitalization, spelling, sentence structure, and word usage.	Almost no errors in punctuation, capitalization, spelling, sentence structure, and word usage.	No errors in punctuation, capitalization, and spelling. No errors in sentence structure or word usage.

Total points possible: 100   **Score and summary comments:**

WHEN SHOULD A SCORING RUBRIC BE USED? WHY USE A SCORING RUBRIC?

When scoring an assignment is likely to be subjective, rubrics are used to improve the objectivity of the scoring process. Rubrics improve the objectivity of scoring by specifying the same criteria and standards to be applied to all students' work. This is especially important when multiple educators will be scoring assignments for different groups of students. The latter half of this book includes examples of assignments when a rubric would be indicated for scoring. Presentations, papers, concept maps, case studies, and portfolios are some of the types of assignments when rubrics should be developed and used for scoring to benefit both the educator and the student. Examples of modifiable analytic rubrics are included in each of these chapters.

Rubrics are most helpful when provided to students before they begin the assignment. Rubrics communicate expectations to improve the clarity of the assignment for students. This results in avoidance of numerous questions about the assignment and improves the quality of the students' work products. When students know the expectations of the assignment, they are more likely to strive to achieve and exceed the expectations. Students should also be encouraged to use the rubric for self-evaluation and revision before submission of the final version to the educator for grading.

Rubrics save time in scoring by clearly specifying levels of performance. This reduces the time required to record what frequently seems like the same thing over and over again with each student. Also, the specificity of the rubric will reduce errors and omissions in scoring and prevents grading assignments inconsistently from the first paper to the last or even student to student. The more specific the rubric, the more consistent the scoring.

Scoring rubrics allow a concise format for providing more descriptive feedback to students. Once completed, the scoring rubric can be pasted to the end of a written assignment or returned separately for presentations. Highlight the level of achievement on each criterion and then add comments with each criterion and/or a summary comment. Audio feedback can also be embedded into the document. Students need and deserve timely and substantive feedback that is more descriptive than a holistic grade or a description as meaningless and asinine as "This is a B paper."

WHAT ARE CRITICISMS OF THE USE OF AN ANALYTIC SCORING RUBRIC?

Some educators argue that grades will be too high if students are told what is expected for an assignment. This criticism is unfounded since the purpose of assignments is learning as well as evaluation. Guiding students to a quality product through the provision of a scoring rubric is beneficial to their overall learning. Another argument against the use of a scoring rubric is that it limits student creativity. Yet students can still be creative while understanding what you as the educator believe is the highest-quality product. Finally, some educators feel that evaluation of student knowledge is impaired by providing the expectation in a rubric. However, the rubric is intended to identify the quality of work product rather than the process, so it does not tell the student what and how to produce the product. Thus, the student must apply his or her knowledge of the content and use of critical thinking to provide the quality work product that is expected.

WHAT ARE THE PARTS OF A SCORING RUBRIC?

The criteria to be rated are arranged in rows in the left-hand column. These are major attributes of the work to be evident in the assignment. The levels of quality/performance are arranged in columns across the top. These levels of quality/performance may be identified as "exceeds expectations," "meets expectations," "barely meets expectations," and "does not meet expectations," or "excellent," "good," "fair," and "poor," or "incompetent," "competent," "proficient," and "expert," as described in Table 4.2. The cells within the table include a description of that criterion at that quality level.

TABLE 4.2   Levels of Quality/Performance Related to the Assignment

Expectations	Quality	Performance	Grade
Exceeds expectations	Excellent	Expert	A
Meets expectations	Good	Proficient	B
Barely meets expectations	Fair	Competent	C
Does not meet expectations	Poor	Incompetent	D or F

HOW DOES ONE DEVELOP A RUBRIC?

The development of a scoring rubric is a process that is perpetual since revision is required, especially after first use but likely after each use. This process is illustrated in Figure 4.1.

Step 1: Reflection

Begin by reflecting on the course student-learning objectives and how this assignment contributes to the demonstration of achievement of those objectives. It is important to consider that if this assignment does not directly relate to a specific course student-learning objectives(s), you should not make the assignment. As stated earlier, this constitutes "busy work."

Your reflection continues with determination of the criteria of the assignment and how significant each criterion is to the overall success of the assignment. If you are working with other educators on a course and they will also be using this rubric, it is important that you

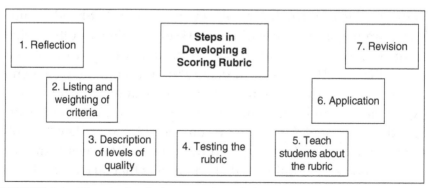

FIGURE 4.1   Steps in developing a scoring rubric.

are all in agreement regarding these criteria and the weighting of the criteria. These decisions reflect your values, such as how important you feel adherence to APA or professional writing is to the overall quality of the work, so there should be a consensus among the educators using this rubric or it will likely not be applied consistently.

Step 2: Listing and Weighting of Criteria

List the essential criteria for evaluation of the assignment. Depending on the assignment, it is likely that there will be 5 to 10 criteria. For example, a paper assignment might include criteria of APA style, professional writing and grammar, references and use of best evidence, and then required content areas. A presentation would involve different criteria such as verbal presentation, visual presentation, references and use of best evidence, audience engagement, and required content areas. Avoid overlapping criteria since there should not be point loss in more than one criterion for the same error or omission. An example of this double jeopardy would be deducting points from Use of Scientific Evidence criterion for not citing research articles AND from References criterion for not having research articles.

Now, consider how important each of these criteria is to the overall success of the assignment for substantiation of achievement of the student-learning objectives. This will determine the weight of the criterion. For instance, consider that one criterion is 5% of the total or a weight of 1. If you consider another criterion to be twice as important as the first criterion, this one would be 10% of the total, or a weight of 2. Finally, determine how many points to assign to this assignment. It is generally easier overall to choose 100 so that it can easily be represented as a percentage, but that is not absolutely necessary. You will find that you will likely need to adjust your point totals and ranges. Use Table 4.3 to list your criteria and the weight of each criterion.

Step 3: Description of Levels of Quality/Performance

Decide how many levels of quality/performance are most appropriate. You would have two for a pass/fail assignment, with one column for "meets expectations" and one column for "does not meet

TABLE 4.3 Weighting of Criteria

Criterion	Weight or Percentage for This Criterion
Total Points:	100%

expectations." You might decide that at least 70% of the criteria must have been scored as "meets expectations" to pass the assignment. If it is an assignment that will receive a point grade, decide if you want to describe three or four levels for each criterion. Either way, the "does not meet expectations" point assignment would be less than 70% of the total points or less than the lowest passing percentage at your school. If you are using only three levels, the "meets expectations" point assignment would be approximately 70% to 85% of the total points, and the "exceeds expectations" point assignment would approximately 86% to 100% of the total points for that criterion. If you are using four levels, the "barely meets expectations" point assignment would be 70% to 79% of the total points, the "meets expectations" point assignment would be 80% to 89% of the total points, and the "exceeds expectations" point assignment would be 90% to 100% of the total points for that criterion.

Determine how your columns will be ordered, from lowest to highest or highest to lowest. The "exceeds expectations" column can either be on the left or the right, depending on what you think is most logical. Since we do read from left to right, you may think that the right column should be the "exceeds expectations" column since the descriptions indicate improvement from left to right. However, you may think that the "exceeds expectations" column should be presented first.

Probably the most difficult task in developing a scoring rubric is describing the quality/performance level of each criterion. Start by describing the characteristics of the "exceeds expectations" level of the criteria and the "does not meet expectations" level of the criteria. Intermediate levels can then be described by considering what errors or omissions would prevent a product from being at that exceptional level and what inclusions could at least partially redeem a very poor work product/performance. Another way to approach this difficult task if you have used this assignment before is to use samples of previous work to identify what qualities made the exceptional work products or performance exceptional. These are descriptions for the "exceeds expectations" level. What omissions or errors were present in the poor work products or performance? These are descriptions for the "does not meet expectations" level. Another consideration is to look at descriptors used in an existing rubric, including the rubrics in this book, and revise these to adapt them for your assignment. Continue to develop your rubric in the rubric template (Table 4.4)

Consider using an online tool to assist you in putting the information in rubric form. Two free web tools are RubiStar (rubistar.4teachers .org/index.php) and iRubric (www.rcampus.com/indexrubric.cfm).

Step 4: Testing the Rubric

Since the scoring rubric is actually a measurement tool, you want to ensure validity and reliability of the tool. Validity refers to the extent to which a tool measures what it is intended to quantify. So, in the case of an evaluation tool such a scoring rubric, validity is whether it measures the specified domain, knowledge, or skill. The act of selection of criteria by an expert or a panel of experts, such as the educators involved in this course, is one step in establishing validity. You should also consider asking another experienced educator who is knowledgeable about the course content to review and critique the assignment description and the rubric.

Reliability is the degree to which a tool produces stable and consistent results. Since rubrics are frequently used by multiple educators or teaching assistants, establishing interrater reliability is very important in refining the rubric. Have all possible scorers use the rubric to score the same paper. Next, conference and identify areas with lack of clarity that contributed to any inconsistent

TABLE 4.4 Rubric Template

Criterion	Does Not Meet Expectations	Nearly Meets Expectations	Meets Expectations	Exceeds Expectations	Student Points for This Criterion
___ (Number of points possible for this criterion)	< ___ points (≤70% of points for this criterion)	___ points (71%–80% of points for this criterion)	___ points (81%–90% of points for this criterion)	___ points (91%–100% of points for this criterion)	
	Description of unacceptable demonstration of achievement of the criterion	Description of marginally acceptable demonstration of achievement of the criterion	Description of good but not exceptional demonstration of achievement of the criterion	Description of exemplary demonstration of achievement of the criterion	
___ (Number of points possible for this criterion)	< ___ points (≤70% of points for this criterion)	___ points (71%–80% of points for this criterion)	___ points (81%–90% of points for this criterion)	___ points (91%–100% of points for this criterion)	
	Description of unacceptable demonstration of achievement of the criterion	Description of marginally acceptable demonstration of achievement of the criterion	Description of acceptable but not exceptional demonstration of achievement of the criterion	Description of exemplary demonstration of achievement of the criterion	

___ (Number of points possible for this criterion)	< ___ points (≤70% of points for this criterion)	___ – ___ points (71%–80% of points for this criterion)	___ – ___ points (81%–90% of points for this criterion)	___ – ___ points (91%–100% of points for this criterion)
	Description of unacceptable demonstration of achievement of the criterion	Description of marginally acceptable demonstration of achievement of the criterion	Description of acceptable but not exceptional demonstration of achievement of the criterion	Description of exemplary demonstration of achievement of the criterion
___ (Number of points possible for this criterion)	< ___ points (≤70% of points for this criterion)	___ – ___ points (71%–80% of points for this criterion)	___ – ___ points (81%–90% of points for this criterion)	___ – ___ points (91%–100% of points for this criterion)
	Description of unacceptable demonstration of achievement of the criterion	Description of marginally acceptable demonstration of achievement of the criterion	Description of acceptable but not exceptional demonstration of achievement of the criterion	Description of exemplary demonstration of achievement of the criterion

(continued)

TABLE 4.4 Rubric Template (*continued*)

Criterion	Does Not Meet Expectations	Nearly Meets Expectations	Meets Expectations	Exceeds Expectations	Student Points for This Criterion
____ (Number of points possible for this criterion)	< ____ points ($\leq$ 70% of points for this criterion)	____ points (71%–80% of points for this criterion)	____ points (81%–90% of points for this criterion)	____ points (91%–100% of points for this criterion)	
	Description of unacceptable demonstration of achievement of the criterion	Description of marginally acceptable demonstration of achievement of the criterion	Description of acceptable but not exceptional demonstration of achievement of the criterion	Description of exemplary demonstration of achievement of the criterion	
____ (Number of points possible for this criterion)	< ____ points ($\leq$ 70% of points for this criterion)	____ points (71%–80% of points for this criterion)	____ points (81%–90% of points for this criterion)	____ points (91%–100% of points for this criterion)	
	Description of unacceptable demonstration of achievement of the criterion	Description of marginally acceptable demonstration of achievement of the criterion	Description of acceptable but not exceptional demonstration of achievement of the criterion	Description of exemplary demonstration of achievement of the criterion	
Total points possible: 100	**Score and summary comments:**				

scoring. Finally, refine the rubric to reduce or eliminate ambiguities so that all educators and students will be clear about each quality descriptor.

Step 5: Teach Students About the Rubric

In addition to including the rubric in the assignment description, whenever discussing the assignment or answering questions about the assignment, refer students to the rubric. Advocate that the students use the scoring rubric in development of their assignment and for self-evaluation and revision of their work product. The ability to evaluate, edit, and improve their work product is an important learning process. You can also foster collaboration by advocating that students exchange drafts and provide feedback to their peers using the scoring rubric.

Step 6: Application

Now it is time to use the rubric to grade assignments. Highlight the relevant qualities of the student's work or performance that determined your decision to assign one category of quality instead of another. Don't feel compelled to rewrite what the rubric already indicates. Only write comments that are not covered in the rubric. Comments can be added for each criterion and/or a summary comment at the end of the rubric.

Consider copying and pasting the rubric at the end of a written assignment, such as a paper, concept map, or case study. With a presentation, give the student the rubric document with scoring and comments. Some classroom management systems (e.g., BlackBoard) include a rubric application. Scores are automatically entered into the online grade book.

If several educators are using the rubric, compare the range and mean of the student groups graded by each educator and note any lack of consistency. Discuss whether the descriptions need to be more explicit or if the importance of consistency of application of the rubric needs to be emphasized. As you and your colleagues grade the assignments, ask everyone to take note of clarifications and additions that are needed.

Step 7: Revision

Assemble your notes and revise your rubric to improve clarity and consistency for the next time you need to use the rubric. Do not wait, since you will likely not remember issues or problems later. You and your colleagues may have discovered areas of ambiguity that need to be clarified or quality aspects that were omitted. You may have discovered characteristics, errors, or omissions that appear in students' work that you didn't think about when the first rubric was developed. You may also decide to include in the revised rubric some of your most common written comments to students. The rubric will likely be refined after each use so that each new iteration has improved validity and reliability as an evaluation tool.

CONCLUSION

This chapter includes a description of types of rubrics and why and how to use a rubric. Examples of a scoring sheet, a holistic rubric, and an analytic rubric for the same assignment were included to allow a comparison of increasing guidance for educator and student. Also included was a step-by-step process toward the development and use of scoring rubrics by educators and students.

5

Assessment, Evaluation, and Grading

Assessment and evaluation are processes fundamental to planning and measuring student learning. According to McDonald (2014, p. 1), "Assessment is the systematic process of collecting and interpreting information to make decisions about student learning and processes." While assessment data can be qualitative or quantitative, they need to be objective. Such assessment data provide valuable information to the educator regarding the efficacy of learning experiences. Thus, once the student's learning needs are identified, the educator establishes learning objectives and determines the measures and methods for assessment and evaluation of student achievement. Analysis of the data collected, as well as the methods and measures used, promotes valid and reliable evaluation of the student's level of achievement of the learning objective(s). There are two types of evaluation: formative and summative (Oermann & Gaberson, 2014). Formative evaluation is used to identify and facilitate students' progress toward successfully meeting the learning objective(s). The data from formative evaluation are intended to identify knowledge gaps that may exist, so learning experiences can be more specifically focused to promote students' success. It does not contribute to the student's course grade. Formative evaluation methods are also intended to provide the educator with information about the effectiveness of teaching/learning strategies. Summative evaluation is conducted after the student has completed required content that measures the student's level of achievement of the learning objectives (Oermann & Gaberson, 2014). Each summative evaluation is assigned a grade. These summative evaluations ultimately contribute to the student's final course grade.

By the end of this chapter, you will learn how to:

- Differentiate between assessment and evaluation
- Collect data for evaluation
- Evaluate student achievement of the course student-learning objectives
- Select a course of action based on formative or summative evaluation results
- Provide meaningful feedback to students regarding achievement of learning objectives
- Identify barriers to meaningful student evaluation
- Assign student grades reflective of the level of achievement of student-learning objectives
- Consider the ethics of student evaluation

ASSESSMENT AND EVALUATION OF ACHIEVEMENT OF STUDENT-LEARNING OBJECTIVES

Assessment and evaluation provide an essential foundation for the learning process. Bastable (2014) emphasizes that while assessment and evaluation methods may both be the same and involve the collection, summarization, interpretation, and use of data, they differ in purpose and timing. Specifically, assessment data assist the educator in identifying learning needs and progress, and provide direction for learning experiences (e.g., lectures and assignments). Green and Emerson (2007) state that assessment is simply ". . . the collection of student work samples in some form, whether tests, papers, projects or presentations" (p. 496).

Evaluation in the strictest sense is to systematically assign value to something. Evaluation in education is the process of assigning a value to student work products such as tests, papers, presentations, and other assignments, for the purposes of determining the level at which the student achieves the learning objectives (Oermann & Gaberson, 2014). The quality of the evaluation is dependent on the quality of the measures and methods chosen to assess student achievement of objectives and the manner in which the data are collected (Hobson, 1998). The evaluation measures must be congruent with the student-learning objectives for the course as discussed in Chapter 2. In addition, both student and educator must be confident that the student data collected for evaluation are reliable and valid representations of the student's level of achievement of the learning objectives (Cizek, 2009).

Clinical Pearl

Assessment is the systematic collection of data that assist the educator in identifying learning needs and progress, and provide direction for learning experiences.

Evaluation is the process of using these data to either inform the educator or student regarding progress toward achievement of the learning objectives (i.e., formative evaluation) or make a judgment regarding achievement of the objective (i.e., summative evaluation).

TYPES OF EVALUATION

Assessment and evaluation of student learning and progress toward achievement of the course student-learning objectives can occur at any time throughout the course. The evaluation can be formative or summative.

Formative Evaluation

Formative evaluation, also referred to as process evaluation (Figure 5.1), supports the teaching and learning process. It informs the educator and student of student progress toward achievement of the learning objectives and facilitates student learning. Collection of student-specific data related to the student's achievement of the learning objectives for formative evaluation occurs prior to when the student is expected to have achieved the learning objective(s) (Oermann, Yarbrough, Saewert, Ard, & Charaskika, 2009). Use assessment techniques such as questioning, 1-minute papers, the muddiest point, and role play exercises described in Box 5.1 to quickly assess student learning and provide formative evaluation feedback to the student. This feedback is intended to facilitate student learning and is not part of the student's final grade. It is also informative to you, the educator, regarding the effectiveness of the teaching/learning strategies.

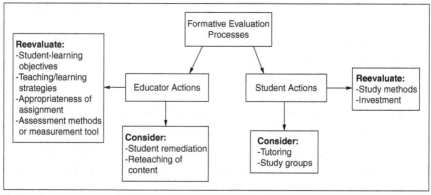

FIGURE 5.1 Formative evaluation processes.

BOX 5.1

Select In-Class Techniques for Formative Evaluation

Questioning	• Ask the student to clarify a concept. (e.g., explain to me how you maintain a sterile field) • Ask the student to compare or contrast (e.g., how are respiratory precautions different from universal precautions?) • Ask for an example (e.g., give an example of reverse isolation)
Muddiest point	• Distribute a 3 × 5 card to each student. Ask the students to identify the "muddiest point" or what seems most confusing or unclear from the learning content.
1-minute paper	• Ask the student to write a brief paper about a specific aspect of the course content or clinical experience. This may be done at the beginning of class so issues can be addressed during that class, or you may want the student to write this immediately before leaving the class and begin the next class with the feedback/ clarification.
Role play	• Divide students into groups of 3 or 4. Have the students create or respond to a created scenario that demonstrates understanding of the content.

Often, the process of evaluation preparation, the evaluation itself, and the review of the findings generated by the evaluation can promote learning and movement toward achievement of the student-learning objectives. In formative evaluation, the student and educator have an opportunity to reflect on the student's progress toward specified learning objectives. Timely and substantive feedback facilitates students' self-awareness of current progress toward achieving the learning objectives, identifies learning gaps that may exist, and raises awareness of learning still required to successfully achieve the course learning objectives (Bastable, 2014). Formative evaluation may yield information or concerns about the student's motivation and investment in the course. Discuss any concerns with the student and explore ways they can be addressed. Remember that formative evaluation is about facilitating the student's success.

Formative evaluation also informs the educator with respect to the learning experiences planned. For example, several strategic questions about required readings can inform the educator of the student's basic knowledge and understanding prior to providing new learning experiences. The educator may use results from formative evaluation throughout the course to adjust the student-learning objectives, planned learning experiences, teaching/learning strategies, or assessment and evaluation methods and measures, in order to better meet the learning needs of the students. These results may indicate that student remediation is necessary, or the content needs to be retaught.

Consider the following situation. You have just finished a class discussing the difference between social and therapeutic communication in health care. You provide a clinical scenario in which both forms of communication are demonstrated. You then ask the students to write a 1-minute paper highlighting the difference between social and therapeutic communication based on the scenario. You review the papers and realize that many of the students in the class are still struggling with differentiating between these two forms of communication. Based on this feedback, you inform the students in the next class that their responses indicate they are not clear on this content. You then review the content and provide additional scenarios for students to practice and discuss.

Note, in this situation, the information gathered was used in a formative manner to direct the learning experience and facilitate student understanding. No grade was given for the 1-minute paper. Consider teaching/learning strategies that you are using and how they provide an opportunity for formative evaluation.

MEANINGFUL FEEDBACK TO STUDENTS

Formative evaluation may show that the student has met the learning objective or is progressing as expected toward the learning objective. The formative evaluation might also show the student is not progressing as expected toward the learning objective or has yet to meet the learning objective. This provides an opportunity for the educator to explore other teaching/learning strategies with the student to better facilitate student learning and success while there is still time to do so. This involves creating a safe learning environment for the student and providing feedback in a manner that is supportive and directive. Educators should provide feedback in a respectful manner that offers hope and facilitates confidence in the student to continue to work toward the learning objectives. Bastable (2014) points out that fear can undermine the evaluation process. For example, there may be fear of failure, fear of disappointing others (including the educator), self-doubt, and lack of self-confidence, which in turn can cause the student to feel very vulnerable. While vulnerability may be exhibited through increased sensitivity, anxiety, and tearfulness, it may also take the form of anger, defensiveness, and blaming. Meaningful, nonjudgmental feedback to the student that is clear, supportive, and directive is essential to facilitating continued learning. A three-step formula for providing feedback includes the following components.

- Acknowledge the student's strengths. Provide positive feedback regarding what the student did well.
- Identify the area(s) for improvement.
- Explore learning strategies to facilitate student learning and success.

For example, consider the following situation reviewing a student's results of a medication pretest. The educator says, "I see that you got all of the medication calculation questions correct. That is a real strength." Next, the educator identifies or asks the student to identify the area(s) presenting the biggest challenge. For a student unable to do this, the educator says, "I see that you really struggled with the content related to side effects of medication." This leads to the discussion with the student as to what the problem may be and how to potentially correct it. The student must be clear on what needs to be done differently in order to meet the learning objective. For example, the educator stating, "It is important that you can describe the major side effects of each of the medications that we cover in class" provides immediate and clear feedback regarding learning still needed with respect to the learning objective. Next, reflect with the student on his or her learning process. Clarify with the student-learning strategies already attempted. As part of this discussion, encourage the student to be as specific as possible in how he or she has attempted to learn the needed content or skill. In some cases, the student may acknowledge that he or she has not fully used the original learning strategies and may recommit to do so. The student may be unaware of not implementing the suggested learning strategy as intended. This is an opportunity for clarification of the learning strategy. For example, a student may report studying, but further exploration reveals the student simply highlighted information while reading and reviewed by reading highlighted information without reflection on his or her own comprehension. A student consistently using recommended learning strategies, however, may need alternative learning strategies. Clarifying with the student other learning strategies being used helps avoid a situation where potential alternative learning approaches suggested by the educator are met with, "I've already tried that." Once current methods for learning have been clarified, explore alternative learning strategies or methods that may be helpful for the particular area of difficulty. This process enables the student to safely reflect on his or her progress and actively engage in the learning process.

The variety of available technology expands the means by which feedback can be provided. Audio feedback, in which you record your feedback for the student, can be more time efficient and has the added benefit of capturing inflections in tone that are not as easily conveyed in the written word. Feedback can be given via video conferencing individually as well as in groups. Videotaping broad feedback to a class where similar issues are identified across the board can be an effective strategy to give feedback in a manner that everyone hears the same information at the same time and saves valuable class time.

Clinical Pearl

Meaningful feedback to students is respectful, clear, hopeful, supportive, and directive. A basic formula for meaningful feedback to students includes:

- Acknowledging the student's strengths
- Clearly identifying areas for improvement
- Exploring and agreeing on specific learning strategies to facilitate student success

There are occasions when conducting a formative evaluation where the student is determined to be at risk of not successfully being able to meet the learning objectives of the course. It is imperative to discuss this with the student to provide the opportunity to make an informed decision about how to progress in the course or to withdraw from the course. A student at risk may need specific tutoring related to the course and learning objectives. It is helpful to have potential tutors identified if this is an option for the student. Students who are progressing successfully toward meeting the learning objectives in the course, or students who successfully completed the course, may serve as effective tutors. You might also encourage the student to attend or create a study group for peer support and assistance in the learning process. Use Exercise 5.1 to explore the provision of feedback in select situations.

Exercise 5.1: Formative Feedback Practice

Identify how you would provide meaningful formative feedback to the student in the following situations.

Situation	Student Strengths	Areas for Improvement	Potential Remedial Teaching/Learning Strategies
You witness a student giving a flu injection. The student has difficulty locating the landmarks on the patient and recaps the needle following giving the injection. You are concerned because this is a skill that the student is expected to perform proficiently by now in this clinical rotation.			
You receive a paper from a graduate student with multiple American Psychological Association (APA) and grammatical errors, though the paper demonstrates excellent use of best evidence and critical thinking.			
Create your own scenario			

SUMMATIVE EVALUATION

Summative evaluation reflects the outcome of the teaching/learning experience that occurred with respect to student learning and level of achievement of the learning objectives (Figure 5.2). The assumption with summative evaluation is that the learner received all the course content and/or proper time to practice the skills required to successfully achieve the associated or relevant learning objectives of the course prior to being evaluated. These evaluations can occur throughout the course wherever a grade is awarded for the unit or

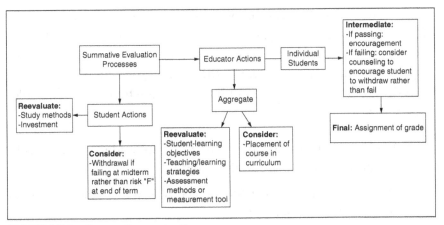

FIGURE 5.2   Summative evaluation processes.

module work that has been completed (Bastable, 2014). Summative evaluation may take the form of a midterm or final examination, a synthesis paper, a presentation, project, or other assignment where the student demonstrates the level of achievement of the learning objectives and a grade is assigned. Each grade assigned contributes to the overall course grade. Data should be collected through clearly identified measures (e.g., test, analytic scoring rubrics) that indicate the level of student achievement of the course learning objectives, and contribute to the final course grade (Cizek, 2009). Data should also be collected throughout the course at intervals that allow students to have a clear understanding of their ongoing success in meeting the course objectives. Based on this understanding, students are able to continue or revise study methods as well as reflect on investment in the course and reinvest in the course as needed. On occasion, a student at likely risk of failing the course may elect to withdraw from the course. Recognizing that withdrawal late in a course can be financially costly as well as result in this being a part of the student's permanent transcript, it is prudent to conduct meaningful summative evaluation and feedback prior to the deadlines established by the university. The final outcome of summative evaluations throughout the course is determination and assignment of a course grade that reflects the level at which the student was able to meet the learning objectives for the course.

Review of all of the summative evaluations collectively for a class of students, that is, aggregate summative data, can be helpful for the educator in determining efficacy of the learning experiences with respect to student achievement of the learning objectives. Questions for reflection include, but are not limited to, the following (Bastable, 2014; Cizek, 2009):

- Were there learning objectives that the students collectively seemed to know prior to the course?

- Were there specific learning objectives with which students had the most difficulty?

- Did the evaluation measures and methods provide an accurate reflection of student achievement of learning objectives? The educator may look at the method whereby the evaluation data were gathered and determine the following.

  - Were the questions on the multiple-choice exam reliable and valid?

  - Did the multiple-choice questions speak to the learning objectives?

  - What was the reliability of the test and various test items?

  - Did the method for evaluation truly reflect achievement of established objectives?

  - Did the rubric (as discussed in Chapter 4 and Part II of this book) effectively measure the specified student-learning objectives?

  - Were the rubrics consistently applied across all students and by all evaluators?

Your responses to these questions can be particularly useful in the postdelivery (after completion of the course) course evaluation as the educator reviews the student-learning objectives, teaching–learning strategies, assignments, assessment, and methods of evaluation for the course. In addition, review of the aggregate summative evaluation data can be helpful when considering course sequencing and in program evaluation and revision.

Clinical Pearl

Summative evaluation is any evaluation of student achievement of the learning objectives that contributes to the student's final course grade.

Review of summative evaluation data collectively, aggregate summative data, can be helpful in course evaluation and revision, course sequencing, and program evaluation.

GRADING STUDENT ACHIEVEMENT
OF LEARNING OBJECTIVES

Green and Emerson (2007) describe grading as "the process by which the *(student)* work is assigned some code—usually A through F or a percentage—that represents the overall quality of the work" (p. 497). The final grade for a course reflects the level at which the student achieved the learning objectives of a course. Walvoord and Anderson (1998) emphasize more broadly that grading serves multiple purposes. They state that in addition to evaluating the level of student achievement of the learning objectives, the grade communicates this to the student as well as to others (e.g., employers, educators) who may review the grade. The grade, and means by which the grade is obtained, is of great interest to the student and provides motivation and organization for the student as he or she progresses toward achievement of the learning objectives. The course grade is a lasting outcome of the teaching/learning experience and both you and the student want to ensure that the grade is an accurate reflection of the student's level of achievement.

The final course grade is the culmination of all summative evaluations, and is calculated as delineated in the evaluation plan for a course. The evaluation plan identifies each component that contributes to the summative grade. The component includes examinations and other assignments. The importance (i.e., weight) of each component of the final grade is reflected by the percentage assigned to that component for the summative grade. Consider the sample evaluation plan with weighted components in Box 5.2. Each component (assignment) that contributes to the summative grade is identified in the first column. The weight of each component with respect to the total score is indicated in the second column. The grade earned by the student on the assignment is identified in the column labeled Percentage Score. Thus on the Discussion Board assignment, which is worth 15% of the student's total grade, the student earned a 90%. This is converted to the weighted score by multiplying 15 x 90 and dividing the sum (i.e., 1350) by 100. Thus, the weighted score is 13.5. After each weighted score is calculated, they are added together to determine the total score earned for the course.

BOX 5.2

Sample of Weighted Evaluation Plan and
Calculated Summative Grade

Component	Weight	Percentage Score	Weighted Score
Discussion Board	15%	90	13.5
Midterm	15%	85	12.7
Major Paper	25%	92	23.0
Portfolio	10%	95	9.5
Concept Map	10%	90	9.0
Comprehensive	25%	89	22.25
Total Score			**90.2%**

A summative grade is also a reflection of how the course was designed, and what content and elements are seen as most important. Essential components of a good grading system include reliability across graders; consistency in feedback; validity; transparency; and sensitivity to differentiation between the levels at which the learning objectives are met, meaningful, and practical (Green & Emerson, 2007). Consider the following questions in evaluating your grading system (Cizek, 2009):

- **Are the measures for the student-learning objectives valid?**

  How do you know that the measures for the student-learning objectives are truly measuring the essential knowledge that is needed? A valid measure is one that is measuring what you are intending to measure. As the educator and the content expert, it is your responsibility to evaluate the validity of the measures and methods of evaluation you have incorporated in your course. Educators with similar areas of expertise can serve as experts in providing feedback on the content validity of the measures. Review measures to ensure that successful achievement of the measure actually reflects the student-learning objectives. If the learning objective requires that the student identify risk factors for heart disease, then a multiple-choice test question in which the student identifies those risk factors would be a valid test item. However, if the learning objective requires the student to synthesize the recent literature about risk factors for heart disease in children, a multiple-choice question would not be a valid measure because the ability to synthesize the literature is not being measured.

- **Is there a plan for ensuring interrater reliability?**

  Interrater reliability refers to the consistency among those grading the same assignments. For example, if more than one person is grading an assignment, a system should be in place to check and ensure that each grader is using the same criteria and is grading the assignment the same way. Despite who does the grading, the score or the grade should be similar. A clearly written scoring rubric is one way to ensure that this happens. It is preferable to have the individuals using the scoring rubric be a part of its development. However, that may not be logistically possible or a previously designed rubric may be used. Regardless, the use of any rubric that is being used among graders should be evaluated. A simple strategy is to have graders grade several of the same assignment and review the grade and feedback for consistency. If there are differences, the graders need to determine why there were differences and come to consensus regarding how the assignments will be graded to ensure intergrader consistency.

- **Is there consistency in feedback to the student with respect to grades and how they were determined?**

  Clearly establish and communicate the criteria for the assignment and the grading process at the beginning of the course. This can be done in the syllabus or through the use of an assignment description or rubric that clearly delineates assignment expectations. Specific feedback regarding how the learning objectives were met or not met should be provided to the student.

- **Are grades transparent in that the students know exactly what the course objectives are and how they will be measured?**

  The grading should be able to differentiate between different levels of achievement. Someone who does a fair job should not have the same grade as someone who does an excellent job. Well-constructed rubrics with levels of differentiation assist with this aspect of the grading process and aid in the prevention of grade inflation.

- **Is the grading system made of meaningful components?**

  The assignments and required student work and time investment should have meaning and value to the individuals who are taking the course. Are the assignments relevant to the student-learning objectives and content being learned? Are the assignments designed so that essential knowledge of the course required to meet the learning objectives can be demonstrated by the student? Do the assignments have practical relevance in that the student will need to utilize this knowledge in his or her professional role?

- **Is the grading system practical?**

  Can the grading system be easily implemented and carried out? Are rubrics developed and used? Is the time spent in grading realistic and consistent with the importance and weighting of the assignment?

Walvoord and Anderson (1998) emphasize that effective grading processes are built on the premise that student learning is the primary goal. Students want to be successful. Involving the student in the learning and grading process is essential. The educator's purpose is to teach and provide the expectations, information, motivation, and resources to facilitate student success.

ETHICS OF EVALUATION AND GRADING

As educators, our charge is to facilitate learning for the student in a manner that is ethical and equitable. As part of that responsibility, we have ethical responsibility to the student related to evaluation and grading (Martinson, 2009). Guidelines or strategies to ensure that we are ethical in our evaluation and grading practices include that we establish and clearly communicate the course expectations/learning objectives and criteria by which these learning objectives will be measured to the student at the beginning of the course. A well-constructed scoring rubric provided to the student at the beginning of the course can aid in this process.

Once the summative evaluation is complete, students should be assigned the grade they earned. The grade is based on the student's level of achievement of the learning objectives as demonstrated through evaluation of their performance on the measures initially communicated to the student (Martinson, 2009). The grade should not be adjusted up or down based on personal preferences or as a favor to students. While this seems obvious, situations do arise where the student requests a change in his or her grade. Keep in mind, if an adjustment is made in one student's grade then that adjustment should be consistently applied to the remaining students, and the rationale shared with the class. Practices such as curving grades, rounding grades up, and giving extra-credit points undermine the reliability and validity of the student's grade and the learning process. They also undermine the quality of the nursing program. Most importantly, however, the ultimate concern is that these adjustments allow a potentially unsafe clinician to continue in the program and become a risk to patients.

Grading is a process that can be challenged publically, through academic and legal processes. Legal defensibility refers to the ability of a grade to "withstand legal challenges" (Pope, 2007, p. 4). Clarity and transparency in grading processes minimize confusion about the final grade earned by the student, strengthen trust between the educator and student, and decrease the likelihood that a final grade will be challenged. However, in the event a grade is challenged, a clearly designed and communicated evaluation plan that incorporates reliable, valid, and objective measures of student achievement of course learning objectives provides evidence to support the grade earned and assigned.

CONCLUSION

This chapter provided a discussion regarding assessment and evaluation of the student's achievement of learning objectives. Formative and summative evaluations were defined and the purpose and implications for educator and student actions were discussed. Barriers to meaningful evaluation along with strategies and considerations for providing meaningful feedback to students were explored. Perspectives and considerations with respect to the meaning and process of grading assignments and assigning a course grade were reviewed. Finally, ethical considerations for evaluation and grading were discussed.

6

Papers

Educators frequently use papers as written assignments throughout the curriculum for evaluation of student achievement of learning objectives (Bickes & Schim, 2010; Hobson, 1998; LaRocco, 2010; Oermann, 2013; Oermann & Gaberson, 2014; Svinicki & McKeachie, 2011). Papers are a vehicle for professional communication that require presentation of original, scholarly learning through a working knowledge of grammar, sentence structure, format, and style (Roberts & Goss, 2009). Writing papers is a skill and an art. Oermann and Gaberson (2014) emphasize ". . . writing is a developmental process that improves with practice" (p. 168). Papers can vary in scope, focus, complexity, and presentation and thus are categorized as major and minor paper assignments. A major paper is distinguished from a minor paper by the increased depth and complexity required for successful completion (Griffin & Novotny, 2012). Examples of major paper assignments include complex clinical reviews, evidence-based project reports, and research papers; whereas minor papers typically include shorter written assignments such as essays and narratives. Other written assignments such as case studies, concept maps, and reflective journals are subjects of future chapters. This chapter focuses on major papers and essay-type minor paper assignments for evaluation of student-learning objectives.

By the end of this chapter, you will learn how to:

- Describe reasons to use papers for evaluation

- Differentiate between major and minor written paper assignments

- Design a clear assignment description for major and minor papers

- Identify prerequisite knowledge and/or resources required by students for major and minor papers

- Develop or adapt a scoring rubric for major and minor papers

USING MAJOR AND MINOR PAPER ASSIGNMENTS FOR EVALUATION

Educators use paper assignments to evaluate the achievement of student-learning objectives (Bickes & Schim, 2010; Hobson, 1998; LaRocco, 2010; Oermann, 2013; Oermann & Gaberson, 2014; Svinicki & McKeachie, 2011). Well-designed paper assignments provide students with the opportunity to demonstrate the achievement of higher-level cognitive learning objectives that require analysis, evaluation, or creation. Paper assignments that require students to conceptualize or synthesize the information help support students' achievement of affective learning objectives. The purpose of the paper assignment needs to be clearly linked to the student-learning objectives. The use of papers as an assignment for evaluation also facilitates students' intellectual growth (Fallahi, Wood, Austad & Fallahi, 2006); critical thinking skills, professional communication skills, and professional identity (Roberts & Goss, 2009); problem-solving skills and clinical judgment (Oermann & Gaberson, 2014); and self-efficacy (Shatzer et al., 2010).

Major Paper Assignments

A major paper is a written assignment that requires the student to produce original, scholarly work. Oermann (2014, p. 169) emphasizes, "Through these written assignments, students develop an understanding of the content they are writing about, and they learn how to communicate their ideas in writing." Major papers typically reflect a review and use of primary scholarly literature sources that are analyzed and synthesized into the paper. While length alone is not a primary determinant, a major paper is typically longer than a minor paper due to the additional content that is required. Typically a major paper requires a significant investment of student preparation time and energy to write, and thus should be a relevant and meaningful learning experience and should contribute to a larger portion of the student's final grade than a minor paper. Types of major papers often assigned are described in Table 6.1.

TABLE 6.1 Types of Major Paper Assignments

Assignment	Description
Comprehensive clinical paper	Focus on the medical condition of a patient and application of care required, review and application of relevant literature to inform the clinical situation, enhance student understanding, and explore implications for application in future clinical situations.
Integrative literature review	"A synthesis of published studies to answer questions about a phenomenon," issue, or concept (Schmidt & Brown, 2012, p. 279).
Systematic literature review or synthesis paper	A rigorous, systematic synthesis of research findings, published and unpublished, about an issue, concept, or phenomenon (Schmidt & Brown, 2012). Includes a clearly identified method for obtaining the literature to be reviewed and the process for reviewing the literature. May be assigned as a stand-alone major paper or may be part of a larger written assignment such as an evidence-based practice project or research paper.
Analysis paper	A paper in which a concept, theory, strategy, or situation is examined to facilitate understanding (Walker & Avant, 1995).
Critical analysis paper	"A paper in which students analyze issues, compare options and develop arguments for a position" (Oermann, 2013, p. 197).

(continued)

TABLE 6.1   Types of Major Paper Assignments (*continued*)

Assignment	Description
Evidence-based practice (EBP) reports	EBP papers are often culminating major papers that focus on the development and implementation of an EBP project; they may be developed and written over several semesters.
Research proposal or paper	Research proposals provide the rationale, supportive background literature, goals, and aims for proposed research. The research question(s) or hypothesis, along with the proposed research design and methods planned, are thoroughly described. A list of references that were used is included along with an appendix where specific forms used in the research study can be viewed. Often there is a required format that is institution specific for research proposals. Research papers are often culminating major papers that may be developed and written over several semesters. In addition to the above information, they include a review of the research data generated and analyzed, a discussion of the findings, and conclusions.
Journal article	A manuscript developed according to the identified publisher's guidelines with the purpose of being submitted for publication.

Require students to write in accordance with guidelines set forth in the most current *Publication Manual of the American Psychological Association* (APA). The basic structure of a major clinical paper is outlined in Box 6.1. Specific academic settings often provide the format for major research or project papers, and those specific rules must be followed in order for the student to progress.

Minor Paper Assignments

Despite its name, a minor paper is no less important than a major paper as a written assignment used for evaluation. Minor papers reflect scholarly learning and can be used for formative as well as summative evaluation. Minor papers can be distinguished from major papers in that they tend to be more focused and are not expected to have the depth of major papers. Extensive literature review is typically not expected for minor papers although referencing of sources may be necessary. Minor papers are not intended to require a large investment of student time and energy and, as such, contribute a lower percentage to the final grade when used for summative evaluation.

BOX 6.1

Basic Structure of a Major Clinical Paper

Title Page	Title concisely communicates the main idea of the paper (12 words or less) Includes author's name and name of organization
Abstract (optional)	Provides a concise summary of the paper Includes major sections as prescribed in the APA manual and one or two sentences about each
Introduction/ background information	Introduces the clinical situation or problem Summarizes current literature regarding the clinical situation or issue Includes what is known, theoretical understandings, and how this relates to the focus of the patient care
Content	Describes the clinical situation and care that was provided
Discussion	Discusses the clinical issue/problem and care with respect to the literature reviewed Includes how the literature informs the clinical situation Includes strengths and weaknesses
Conclusion	Includes the following: • A summary of what was learned • What questions remain • The implications for the future • Next steps
Summary	Provides an overview of what was covered in the paper
References	Includes cited scholarly sources

Examples of minor papers include worksheets that you ask students to complete related to their readings, concept maps, case studies, journal entries, critical appraisals, and essays. An essay is a short paper that has a specific focus. It is usually no longer than five pages with few or even no references. The format is usually an introduction, body, and then conclusion. Common essay assignments are a philosophy of nursing paper early in an undergraduate curriculum, a reaction paper to the first clinical experience for undergraduates, a career plan paper during an undergraduate senior course, and short essays on various topics during graduate programs.

Clinical Pearl

Equally important, major and minor papers provide the student an opportunity to demonstrate achievement of higher-level student-learning objectives.

WRITING THE ASSIGNMENT DESCRIPTION

The most important aspect of the assignment description is the purpose of the paper and the relationship of the purpose to the course objectives. Clearly identify the expectations for the paper assigned and focus the student toward achievement of the specific learning objectives. Most likely you will ask students to do a paper related to a key content area of the course. Students may write a paper on the same topic or theme. In situations where students select their own topic, it is helpful to have a list of possible topics for student selection to avoid duplication. If students determine their own topic, have a process for the educator to review and approve the topic. This avoids situations in which the student, with good intentions, selects a topic that will not meet the expected learning objectives of the paper assignment. Provide a deadline for the topic approval and provide students with timely and substantive feedback.

Be specific and realistic about the expected page limit and what you expect to be accomplished within that page limit. While students may be concerned about exceeding the page limit, a paper that is too short is unlikely to have achieved the purpose of the paper or include essential elements. Also, be specific about formatting (Table 6.2). While you will likely want papers in APA format, consider specifying whether an abstract is required. As previously discussed, a major paper will most likely require an abstract, while an abstract of an essay that is three to five pages is unlikely to be helpful for the writer or the reader. Remind students that APA is double spaced and 12-point font. The recommended font is Times New Roman but another serif font can be used. Students will sometimes change the font style or size to be within the page limit, so be specific in the assignment description.

TABLE 6.2   Comparison of Major and Minor Paper Assignments

	Major Paper	Minor Paper
Purpose	Typically addresses several of the student-learning objectives of the course	Typically addresses one particular student-learning objective
Focus	Broad, complex issues to be addressed in depth	Specific, variable depth
Structure	APA format and style; may have multiple headings and sections	Alternative formats linked specifically to the setting and assignment. May or may not require a title page, abstract, or reference list
Length	Variable; 10–20 pages; (a thesis or dissertation may exceed 100 pages)	1–5 pages
Time to complete	Several weeks	Minutes to several days
References	Required; reflect scholarly sources	Varies with the assignment. However, if sources are used, they should be acknowledged
Setting	Individual assignment Completed outside the classroom	Variable; individual or group assignment, which may be completed in a classroom, clinical, or outside setting
Delivery method	Electronic delivery through assignment management system in a reviewable format Submitted through antiplagiarism software	Variable; may be hand delivered or electronic depending on the assignment
Grade	Greater percentage of the weighted grade	Lower percentage of the weighted grade

Clearly explain whether you require scholarly references for the paper assignment. Major papers will most likely require scholarly references. Depending on the topic and purpose of a minor paper, you may or may not want to require references. If this is a reaction paper or an essay about the student's opinion, it is likely you will not want references since it will increase the chance that you get someone else's opinion rather than the student's opinion or reaction. For an evidence-based paper, you will want references. Students find it helpful when the number and type of references expected are identified in the assignment description.

Specify how and when the paper is due. Most likely you will want an electronic version, which allows you to use track changes and comment when you are giving feedback. Specify the file type, which is most likely Word, and how you want the file named, such as LASTNAMEESSAY.docx or LASTNAMEPAPER.docx. Caution the student against submitting a PDF document, as you will not be able to use track changes to add feedback and comments. Clearly identify where you want the student to submit the electronic version of the paper. Most frequently this is either via the assignment manager in your learning management system or by e-mail. Papers submitted to the educator's e-mail can take up a lot of space, and depending on the volume of e-mail received can be easily overlooked.

Clinical Pearl

Be specific in the assignment description. The more specific you are, the fewer e-mails you will receive for clarification. Encourage students to carefully review the assignment description and rubric and use them to evaluate their own paper prior to submission.

Plagiarism can be prevented in a number of ways. First, discuss what plagiarism is and that even unintentional plagiarism is plagiarism. Provide educational materials about academic dishonesty and consider having students sign an honor statement. Ask for the paper in stages, which makes it more difficult for a student to submit a purchased paper. Finally, ask students to submit their paper to antiplagiarism software (e.g., Turnitin) websites, which can check the paper for originality. This software can be set up so that a student has an opportunity to review the originality report of the paper prior to the final submission of the paper. For detection, the educator can submit the paper through the antiplagiarism software. If the report indicates that the paper submitted by the student is not the student's own work, review the paper and details of the report for accuracy (Anderson, 2009). If you do not have access to antiplagiarism software, consider submitting suspect phrases in quotation marks into a search engine to see if that exact phase can be found. Also, look at the properties of a paper to determine the original author of the paper. Remember that you will be that author if you did give the student a template. If you do suspect plagiarism, follow institutional policies. Most universities have an academic integrity council that makes rules regarding plagiarism and it is not the role of the educator to determine intent.

Clinical Pearl

Prevent plagiarism by ensuring that students know what it is and is not, providing education on ways to prevent even unintentional plagiarism, requiring students to sign an honor statement, asking for papers in stages, and requiring students to submit their papers to an antiplagiarism software program so that they can detect and correct any unintentional plagiarism.

Detect plagiarism using antiplagiarism software, search engines using exact phrases that are suspicious, and looking at the properties for the original author.

ALWAYS report plagiarism and other instances of academic dishonesty.

IDENTIFYING PRIOR KNOWLEDGE AND/OR RESOURCES TO BE AVAILABLE FOR STUDENTS

Students need resources on APA style for their references. If you do not require that they buy the APA manual, you may consider providing the URL for Owl Purdue Online Writing Lab (owl.english.purdue.edu/owl/resource/560/01/) in the assignment description.

Students may also need resources on professional writing. There is a tremendous range of writing skills within our student groups and much of this is dependent upon high school English and/or composition courses and their past experience in professional writing. Consider how many writing assignments the student has had before this course and whether the student received valuable feedback on those assignments. You may be surprised by the limited writing skills of even graduate students, but if the student graduated from a college with very large nursing classes, it is unlikely that writing assignments were common. *The Elements of Style* (Strunk & White, 2000) is a classic, easy-to-use reference on commonly misunderstood rules of usage and composition. In addition, here are some valuable websites to include in your assignment description.

- Owl Purdue Online Writing Lab: www.libertyguide.com/resources/ways-to-improve-your-professional-writing-skills
- UCLA Graduate Writing Center: gsrc.ucla.edu/gwc/resources/grammar-punctuation-style-and-usage.html
- Grammar Girl: www.quickanddirtytips.com/grammar-girl
- GrammarBook.com: www.grammarbook.com

Provide information about plagiarism and ways to detect unintentional plagiarism. There are many excellent websites that can provide your students with this crucial information.

- Indiana University School of Education: www.indiana.edu/~istd/definition.html
- Acadia University Tutorial regarding Plagiarism: library.acadiau.ca/tutorials/plagiarism
- Plagiarism.org: www.plagiarism.org/plagiarism-101/what-is-plagiarism
- University of Southern Mississippi (includes quizzes): www.lib.usm.edu/legacy/plag/plagiarismtutorial.php

Clinical Pearl

Find great web resources to share with your students but check the links every semester to ensure that the link is not broken and that the web resource is still current.

Most colleges have a writing center to support students. Consider including information on how to access writing assistance in your syllabus. Usually there is an actual center on campus and a virtual center online. Keep in mind that the purpose of these centers is to assist the student in rewriting and revising their paper; they will not rewrite the paper for the student.

MODIFYING FOR ONLINE DELIVERY

While there is no modification necessary for this assignment, you should be very specific about how you want the paper delivered, such as through the assignment manager of the learning management system or as an email attachment. Also, as previously described, be specific about how you want the file to be named.

EVALUATING THE PAPER

Papers can be used for formative and summative evaluation. While major papers are most often used for summative evaluation, at times students will request that their paper be reviewed and feedback given prior to when the paper is due. This can be a very time-consuming process for the educator and may not be realistic depending on the number of students in the class and other responsibilities. Also, while educator feedback given is often helpful and the student revises the paper accordingly, the final paper submitted for a summative grade is then often much higher than it might have been otherwise. Hobson (1998) cautions that this informal review process may undermine the reliability and validity of the grade assigned and contributes toward grade inflation. Dividing a major paper into smaller progressively sequenced writing assignments that build on each other is a method that promotes student success in writing a major paper (Bramer & Basting, 2013; Oermann & Gaberson, 2014). In this case, construction of the major paper is done by sections, which are graded along the way. Feedback on each section, provided by the educator to the student, can be used in rewriting the paper as the sections are combined and the major paper completed.

Smith (2008) reports that students preferred feedback on a scored rubric to include comments of what was done well along with what could be done better. The following rubric (Table 6.3) provides a

TABLE 6.3 Modifiable Scoring Rubric for a Paper Assignment

Criterion (Points Possible)	Does Not Meet Expectations	Nearly Meets Expectations	Meets Expectations	Exceeds Expectations	Score and Comments
	≤7	8	9	10	
APA (10) Title page Headings Citations (if references required) Reference page (if references required) Font, layout, margins	Major problems with implementation of APA style in title page, headings, citations, and/or reference page. Font, layout, and/or margins do not adhere to APA format, which affect overall flow and readability of the paper.	Several errors in title page, headings, citations, reference page, font, layout, and/or margins that are minimal distractions but do not affect overall flow and readability of the paper.	Minimal APA errors in title page, headings, citations, reference page, font, layout, and/or margins that do not distract from the content or readability of the paper.	Consistent adherence to APA criteria in title page, headings, citations, and/or reference page. Font, layout, and/or margins adhere to APA format.	
	<3.5	3.5	4	5	
Introduction (5)	Incomplete or unfocused purpose statement. There is no clear introduction of main topic and/or the structure of the paper is missing.	The introduction does state the paper's purpose but is convoluted and not engaging. The introduction does not clearly state the topic or preview the structure and content of the paper.	The introduction states the paper's purpose in a single sentence but fails to be engaging. The introduction states the main topic but does not adequately preview the structure of the paper.	The introduction clearly and concisely states the paper's purpose in a single sentence that is engaging and thought provoking. The introduction clearly describes and states the main topic and previews the structure and content of the paper.	

	< 3.5	3.5	4	5
Organization/ structure (5)	No evidence of structure or organization. Ideas are not fully developed. Minimal use of transitions throughout the paper.	Logical organization, but some ideas are not fully or consistently developed. Transitions are awkward at times but the flow is adequately maintained.	Writer demonstrates logical sequencing of ideas through well-developed paragraphs; transitions are typically used to enhance organization.	Writer demonstrates logical and subtle sequencing of ideas through well-developed paragraphs; transitions are used to enhance organization.
	≤ 39	40–43	44–59	50–55
Body of paper: required content includes ___ (55)	Much of required content is not developed and the state of clinical evidence is not addressed.	Most required content is developed with background and the current state of the clinical evidence.	Required content is thoughtfully and systematically developed with background and the current state of the clinical evidence.	All required content is thoughtfully and systematically developed and relevant with background and the current state of the clinical evidence.

(continued)

TABLE 6.3 Modifiable Scoring Rubric for a Paper Assignment (*continued*)

Criterion (Points Possible)	Does Not Meet Expectations	Nearly Meets Expectations	Meets Expectations	Exceeds Expectations	Score and Comments
	< 3.5	3.5	4	5	
Conclusion (5)	There is no conclusion.	The conclusion summarizes the contents of the paper.	The conclusion summarizes the contents of the paper but does not effectively summarize the significant conclusions in an interesting manner.	The conclusion reviews the main points of the paper and clearly and effectively summarizes significant conclusions in an interesting manner.	
	≤ 7	8	9	10	
References (if required) (10)	Based on less than five nonresearch references; liberal use of .com websites.	Based on five to seven references with less than three research references and/or use of some .com websites.	Based on eight to ten references with at least three research references; only websites used were .org, .edu, or .gov.	Based on more than ten references with at least three research references; only websites used were .org, .edu, or .gov.	

102

	≤7	8	9	10
Mechanics/usage (10)	Numerous errors in punctuation, capitalization, spelling, sentence structure, or word usage with significant impact on the content and detracts from the paper.	Several errors in punctuation, capitalization, spelling, sentence structure, or word usage with minimal impact on or distraction from the content of the paper.	Few errors in punctuation, capitalization, spelling, sentence structure, or word usage, which do not impact or distract from the content of the paper.	No errors in punctuation, capitalization, or spelling. No errors in sentence structure or word usage.

Total points possible: 100   **Score and summary comments:**

template for grading a paper. It can be modified as needed. Return the electronic version of the paper to the student with comments and track changes, and a copy of the completed rubric pasted at the bottom of it.

CONCLUSION

Major and minor papers are time-consuming for students to complete and educators to grade. Well-defined assignment expectations help the student write a paper that is clearly linked to and meets the expectations for the course student-learning objectives. Clearly designed scoring rubrics are helpful for communication of the quality of the paper expected from the student and provide the educator with a focused and consistent method for evaluation.

7

Presentations

Nurse educators frequently use presentation assignments either as a teaching/learning strategy or as a method of evaluation. This chapter focuses on student evaluation of either individual or student group presentations, which may be delivered either in class or online. Presentations are excellent synthesis assignments and allow students to show innovation and creativity.

By the end of this chapter, you will learn how to:

- Describe reasons to use presentations for evaluation
- Design a clear assignment description for presentations for evaluation
- Identify prerequisite knowledge and/or resources required by students for a presentation assignment
- Adapt a presentation assignment of online courses, including how to use the narration option of PowerPoint
- Discuss best practices for the use of PowerPoint for presentations

- Develop or adapt a scoring rubric for a presentation assignment
- Consider the involvement of students in the peer evaluation of presentations

USING PRESENTATIONS FOR EVALUATION

There are many reasons to make a presentation assignment for either undergraduate or graduate students. Presentations evaluate achievement of objectives in the cognitive and affective domains. However, if the presentation includes a demonstration of a skill, objectives in the psychomotor domain may also be evaluated.

Student learning when doing a presentation begins with a search for pertinent literature. This reinforces how to do a literature search, evaluate the quality of the evidence, and select what is important enough to share with peers. Deep learning of a given topic occurs whether the student chooses or is assigned the topic. The student also develops a sense of ownership of the topic and learns the importance of controlling the learning environment during the presentation.

The process of planning a presentation is a learning experience in project management, especially if this is a group presentation. A project timeline needs to be developed and roles identified. Additionally, if this is a group assignment, the ability to be a productive member of a team will be demonstrated. The importance of communication with team members during the planning process will be appreciated.

The ability to communicate verbally is an important skill, whether communicating to other members of the health care team or making a presentation at a professional meeting. Professionals need communication skills and leaders need exemplary communication skills. Respondents to the Job Outlook 2013 survey by the National Association of Colleges and Employers (2011) rated "ability to verbally communicate with persons inside and outside the organization" and "ability to work in a team structure" as the two most important candidate skills/qualities. Individual presentations focus on this first skill, while group presentations focus on both of these skills.

Unlike a written assignment, a presentation allows students the opportunity to share their work with their student peers. The student practices speaking in a relatively safe environment. The student also learns about presentation software and best practices for use of this software.

Another benefit of assigning presentations is that derived by the other students. Rotenberg (2012) writes that presentations allow students to teach and learn from one another. To encourage students to give attention to the presentations, involve them in peer evaluation of the presenters (Weimer, 2012). Also, consider evaluating comprehension of the presented content through questions or discussion. Students generally give more attention when the answer to "will this be on the exam?" is yes.

Clinical Pearl

Reasons for using a presentation assignment for evaluation include reinforcement of the principles of literature search and review, development of project management skills, and improvement of communication and presentation skills.

When evaluating a presentation, include content as well as delivery. Since an important reason for presentations is the contribution to the learning of the student peers, accuracy of information presented is crucial. Also of note is whether the information presented is current and evidence based. The presentation should include the information that you identify as required and it should be organized in a logical manner. The presentation should include an introduction, body, and conclusion, just as a paper would (Moyer & Wittman-Price, 2008). Instruct students to include references either as the last slide(s) or as a separate document so that student peers can have access to these references if they desire.

WRITING THE ASSIGNMENT DESCRIPTION

The most important aspect of the assignment description is the purpose of the presentation and the relationship of the purpose to the course objectives. Most likely you will ask students to do presentations related to a key content area of the course. If you assign topics, make the assignments public so that students or student groups can avoid overlap and redundancy. If students are to choose a topic, list possible choices. If students are to determine their own topic, include a deadline for submission of the topic for your approval.

If you determine the list of topics or when approving a topic submitted by a student or student group, consider whether that topic can be adequately discussed within the established time limit. When you determine time limits, consider the number of students or student groups in the class and length of time for the class session, allowing approximately 3 to 5 minutes between presentations. For group presentations, it is best to limit the group size to four or five students.

Be clear about the required elements of the presentation; these will also be used in the development of the grading rubric. Depending on the level of student, you might want to specify a typical format for the presentation such as title, objectives, discussion of topic and implications to nursing, significant research if appropriate, summary, and references. You might consider providing a general content outline (Moyer & Wittman-Price, 2008).

Be specific regarding acceptable references and the number of references. If you don't specify a minimum number, students will most likely ask, so do give a recommended number of references. Undergraduate students may need you to clearly exclude Wikipedia as a professional reference and specify which websites types are acceptable. A good guideline is that you will accept .edu, .gov, and .org but you will not accept a .com. Consider identifying how many professional journal articles are required lest the student provide a reference list consisting entirely of websites.

Describe the work products to be submitted prior to the presentation and date and time that these products are due, how the file(s) is to be named, and how the file is to be delivered (i.e., assignment manager of learning management system, Google Docs, e-mail attachment). Specify whether audiovisuals, such as PowerPoint slides, are recommended or required. Specify whether references should be provided on the last slide or as a separate Word document.

It is good practice to ask for major assignments in stages. For undergraduate students, you may ask only for an outline and a list of references for review about 1 week prior to the presentation, and the PowerPoint file the evening before the presentation so it can be posted and made available to classmates. For graduate students, consider asking for an instructional design table (Table 7.1) as a Word document about 1 week prior to the presentation and then the PowerPoint file and a posttest as a Word document the day before the presentation so that they can be posted for classmates. These deadlines prohibit procrastination and the student bringing paper handouts to class. Also, requiring that assignments be submitted in stages also helps to prevent academic misconduct, such as getting presentations from past students or the Internet.

Clinical Pearl

Be VERY specific when writing the assignment description. Describe what should be included in the presentation, what work products are required and when, and the number and types of references required.

TABLE 7.1   Instructional Design Table

| Objectives | Content | Teaching/Learning | |
		Strategies	Evaluation Methods

At the completion of this pre-sentation, the nursing student (or graduate student) will be able to:
• (Objective)
• (Objective)
• (Objective)
• (Objective)
	I. _____
	  A. _____
	  B. _____
	  C. _____
	II. _____
	  A. _____
	  B. _____
	  C. _____
	III. _____
	  A. _____
	  B. _____
	  C. _____
		• (Enhanced lecture/ discussion, case study,etc.)	• (Classroom assessment techniques, posttest,etc.)

IDENTIFYING PRIOR KNOWLEDGE AND/OR RESOURCES TO BE AVAILABLE FOR STUDENTS

Students will need at least basic literature search skills. If they do not have this prerequisite knowledge, then perhaps a professional presentation is not an appropriate assignment or you need to have a tutorial to assist the students in finding, evaluating, and using professional literature. You might consider including the librarian's e-mail address if there is one assigned to nursing students. Students also need resources on American Psychological Association (APA) style for their references. If you do not require that they buy the APA manual, you may consider providing the URL for Owl Purdue Online Writing Lab (owl.english.purdue.edu/owl/resource/560/01) in the assignment description.

Consider posting links to information on presentation skills (such as www.presentationskills.ca; www.youtube.com/watch?v=wh TwjG4ZIJg) and best practices of PowerPoint (such as tep.uoregon .edu/technology/powerpoint/docs/presenting.pdf). A summary of do's and don'ts for PowerPoint is available in Box 7.1. For graduate students who will be writing learning objectives, post links to information on how to write objectives (such as teaching.uncc .edu/articles-books/best-practice-articles/goals-objectives/ writing-objectives-using-blooms-taxonomy).

Clinical Pearl

Find great web resources to share with your students but check the links every semester to ensure that the link is not broken and that it the web resource is still current.

BOX 7.1

Best Practices for PowerPoint

- Do use good contrast such as a dark blue background with white text.

- Do use bullet points rather than complete sentences since you will be tempted to read the complete sentences; do not read your PowerPoint slides to the audience.

- Do restrict the amount of text on slides; use the 6 × 6 rule—no more than 6 lines and no more than 6 words per line.

- Do restrict the number of different fonts in your presentation to two.

- Do use a sans serif font for presentations, such as Arial, Calibri, Berlin Sans, Gill Sans, or Tahoma.

- Do make the text size at least 32 points for headings and 24 points for bullet points.

- Do use illustrations appropriately and sparingly; ask yourself if it really contributes to the presentation. If not, omit it. Avoid .GIF files that repeatedly move and are distracting.

- Do use subtle transitions and animation effects. Headings flying in while spinning are very distracting, but a subtle appear and disappear helps focus on the bullet point being currently discussed.

- Do rehearse; it will likely take approximately 1 minute per slide, so you should not have more than 30 slides for a 30-minute presentation. To ensure that you do not exceed your time limit (and likely cause point loss), rehearse with your slides.

Since the modifiable analytic rubric included in this chapter includes a criterion of active learning, you should include examples of active learning strategies that can be incorporated into a presentation to engage the audience. Moellenberg and Aldridge's (2010) "Sliding away from PowerPoint" is a good reading assignment to encourage the use of PowerPoint as a complement or accessory to the presentation rather than as "the presentation." Avoid the use of "lecture" for a presentation; rather, refer to it as a presentation and the primary method being "enhanced lecture," which incorporates discussion, question, and other classroom assessment techniques on slides, such as matching, completion, short case study.

Information regarding how to deal with presentation anxiety should be shared with students. Encourage the student to use class participation opportunities as opportunities to practice speaking in a group setting. Emphasize preparation and practice in reducing anxiety. Imagery is also advocated; the student should imagine him- or herself delivering an eloquent presentation successfully.

MODIFYING FOR A GROUP PRESENTATION

Just like with individual presentations, group presentations have a preparatory phase and then a delivery phase. During the preparatory phase, the group needs to make assignments and set meeting times. Also, there should be a practice session with all group members participating. If an individual student is not attending meetings or meeting deadlines for group assignments, the group should first try to resolve the issue. If this is unsuccessful, a group meeting with you is required.

For the delivery phase, encourage each group to select a moderator for the presentation. The moderator should introduce the speakers and topics, monitor time, and lead the question-and-answer session. During delivery, the group members should be attentive to the presentations of the other group members (Painter, 2011).

Though you can easily evaluate the actual presentation by each student, it is more difficult to evaluate their overall contribution to the planning and development of the presentation. Consider including a peer evaluation such as Form 3.1, for group members to evaluate their own contribution and the contribution of others in the group. The most significant complaint of students regarding group projects is when a group member does not effectively participate but still gets the grade of the other members who have worked effectively.

MODIFYING FOR ONLINE DELIVERY

To have students do presentations in an online course, you must have a method to visualize both the slides and the presenter, such as Adobe Connect or Blackboard Illuminate. Students must also be able to control advancement of the slides. The educator should have PowerPoint files uploaded and ready for use to limit time loss between presentations.

The alternative to live presentations is to have students narrate a PowerPoint presentation (i.e., voice-over PowerPoint). Instructions (such as Box 7.2) and best practices (www.facultyfocus.com/articles/online-education/adapting-powerpoint-lectures-for-online-delivery-best-practices) need to be provided for students. Since the narrated PowerPoint files are very large, software to compress the file and/or convert to a Flash file (i.e., iSpring) is recommended.

BOX 7.2

Directions for Using the Narration Option in PowerPoint to Make Presentations for Online Delivery

1. Have your PowerPoint developed using bullet points rather than complete sentences (which you would be tempted to read). When deciding how many slides you need, consider that it will generally take you approximately 1 minute per slide assuming you are using the 6 × 6 rule (no more than 6 lines on a slide and no more than 6 words per line).

(continued)

BOX 7.2 *(continued)*

2. Print your notes separately since you will be in slide-show view to record and you will not be able to see notes that you have entered in the notes section. Write yourself notes regarding examples or analogies that you want to use.

3. Click on Slide Show

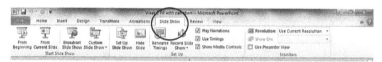

4. Then click on Record Slide Show.

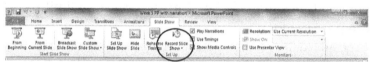

5. Click on Start Recording.

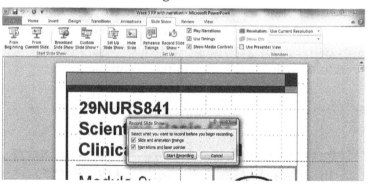

6. You will then see the slide on full screen (slide show view). Talk slowly and clearly. Stop talking at least 2 seconds before you advance the slide. Now wait 2 seconds after advancing the slide before you start to speak again.

7. To stop recording, right click and choose End Show. It takes a little while for embedding all those audio files in the PowerPoint but it will soon go back to normal view.

(continued)

BOX 7.2 (*continued*)

8. You will notice speakers at the bottom right of each recorded slide.

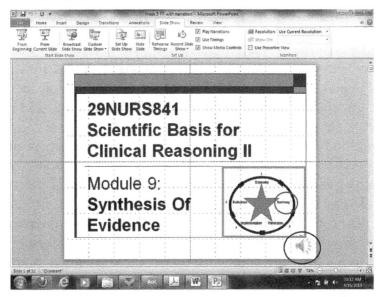

9. If you want to record again, you will be asked if you want to start at the beginning or with the current slide. This way you can update only one slide but make sure you click on End Show before you advance the slide or you will also have to rerecord the next one too.

10. Group presentations in an online class present logistical challenges such as how and when to meet to plan and practice the presentation. Using videoconferencing with Adobe Connect, Blackboard Illuminate, Skype, or Google Hangout for meetings is helpful. An Internet-based scheduling application, such as Doodle (www.doodle.com), can be used to establish best times for meeting and can be set to automatically change to the time zone of the responder. Also, collaborative documents through Google or use of a wiki can allow everyone to add their sections of the presentation and review and provide feedback to other group members.

EVALUATING THE PRESENTATION ASSIGNMENT

In addition to using a grading rubric, you might also include the student audience in the evaluation process. You could simplify the grading rubric or simply ask the students to rate the usefulness of the presentation on a 1 to 10 scale. If you are going to involve students in the evaluation process, it is important that the student peers' and your evaluation criteria be consistent (Rotenberg, 2012).

To allow students to perform a self-evaluation, consider having the presentations recorded. They may think that they did not read from their slides or notecards or that they did not use vocal pauses (e.g., "ah," "umm") as you identified in your evaluation; therefore, it is very helpful for them to be able to view the recording after they receive their grade and scoring rubric.

The following rubric (Table 7.2) can be adapted to include specifics regarding which work products and content you require. Share the rubric with students so they know how they will be evaluated and can plan accordingly. Complete the evaluation rubric either during the presentation or shortly thereafter since you are likely to forget some of the subtleties of the presentation the longer you wait.

TABLE 7.2 Modifiable Scoring Rubric for a Presentation Assignment

Criterion (Points Possible)	Does Not Meet Expectations	Nearly Meets Expectations	Meets Expectations	Exceeds Expectations	Score and Comments
	≤ 14	15–16	17–18	19–20	
Instructional Plan (20) (If Graduate Course)	Multiple weaknesses in instructional plan and objectives not achieved through presentation or instructional plan not submitted by deadline prior to presentation.	Multiple weaknesses in instructional plan or objectives not achieved through presentation.	Objectives not in learned-focused objective form or content outline brief, teaching-learning strategies not identified, evaluation method not identified, presentation was not consistent with plan, or objectives not achieved through presentation.	Objectives in proper form; appropriate content and teaching/learning strategies identified; appropriate evaluation method identified; presentation delivered as planned and objectives achieved.	
	< 3.5	3.5	4	5	
Introduction (5)	Failed to greet audience or introduce self, or qualifications or reason for interest in topic. Did not identify objectives or areas to be discussed.	Failed to greet audience or introduce self, qualifications, or reason for interest in topic. Introduced topic and areas to be discussed but not in objective form.	Greeted the audience. Introduced self but did not identify qualifications or reason for interest. Reviewed objectives in learner-focused measurable form.	Greeted the audience. Introduced self and qualifications to speak on topic. Explained reason for interest in topic. Reviewed objectives listed in learner-focused measureable form.	

(continued)

TABLE 7.2 Modifiable Scoring Rubric for a Presentation Assignment (*continued*)

Criterion (Points Possible)	Does Not Meet Expectations	Nearly Meets Expectations	Meets Expectations	Exceeds Expectations	Score and Comments
	≤ 14	15–16	17–18	19–20	
Discussion of assigned topic with required content (20) (list required content here)	Discussion omitted more than one area of required content. Lack of even basic knowledge of topic evident through presentation and responses to questions. Presentation jumps from topic to topic and impossible to follow.	Discussion did include required content but superficial and/or several inaccuracies noted. Omission of at least one area of required content. Superficial knowledge of topic evident through presentation and responses to questions. Presentation is disorganized and difficult to follow.	Discussion of assigned topic with required content at appropriate depth and detail. Some minor inaccuracies noted. Knowledge of topic is evident through presentation and responses to questions. Presentation is organized.	Exemplary discussion of assigned topic with required content at appropriate depth, detail, and accuracy. Extensive knowledge of topic is clearly evident through presentation and responses to questions. Presentation is organized in an interesting and logical sequence.	

	≤14	15–16	17–18	19–20
Use of scientific evidence (20)	No discussion of the scientific evidence. References list fewer than five references. Multiple errors in APA citations and references.	Limited discussion of scientific evidence related to topic. References list includes at least five to seven references with fewer than three of these research studies. More than two errors in APA citations and references.	Good discussion of scientific evidence related to topic. Reference list includes at least eight references with at least three of these good quality research studies. No more than two errors in APA citations or references.	Exemplary discussion of the scientific evidence related to topic. Reference list includes at least 10 references with at least five good-quality research studies cited. No errors in APA citations or references.

	< 3.5	3.5	4	5
Conclusion/summary (5)	No conclusion or summary. Did not invite questions.	Brief summary with no conclusion or recommendations. Did not invite questions.	Summary of what was discussed but no recommendations given. Invited questions.	Summary of what was discussed and conclusion with recommendations. Invited questions.

(continued)

Criterion (Points Possible)	Does Not Meet Expectations ≤7	Nearly Meets Expectations 8	Meets Expectations 9	Exceeds Expectations 10	Score and Comments
Verbal and nonverbal presentation (10)	Casual attire. Frequent pauses, lots of uhs, hmmms, or you knows, or monotone. Speech is too soft, too loud, too fast, or too slow. Limited vocabulary and frequent mispronunciations. Use of slang or profanity. Almost exclusively reading from slides or notes. Does not look at audience, move, or smile. Distracting mannerisms. More than 20% over time limit.	Casual attire. Hesitancy, some uhs, hmmms, or you knows. Limited variation in intonation. Speech is too soft, too loud, too fast, or too slow. Limited vocabulary and more than two mispronunciations. Use of slang or profanity. Frequently reads from slides or notes. Rarely looks at audience. Stiff body movements. Does not smile. More than 10% over time limit.	Professional attire. No hesitancy or uhs, hmmms, or you knows. Does vary intonation and speech is of appropriate loudness and speed. Good vocabulary and no more than one or two mispronunciations. No use of slang or profanity. Uses notes minimally and does not read from slides. Occasionally looks at audience members. Uses some hand gestures. Smiles when appropriate. No more than 10% over time limit.	Professional attire. Enthusiastic and engaging. Speech is fluid with clear enunciation. Uses voice to communicate interest by varying intonation and appropriate loudness and speed. Excellent vocabulary with no mispronunciations. No use of slang or profanity. No reading from slides. Establishes eye contact with audience; scans room. Natural hand gestures. Smiles when appropriate. Adheres to time limit.	

	≤7	8	9	10
Visual presentation (10)	Many errors in spelling, word usage, or punctuation. Font selection and/or size inappropriate. Use of distracting colors or visuals. Demonstrates no creativity.	More than two errors in spelling, word usage, or punctuation. Font selection and/or size inappropriate. Distracting colors or poor contrast. Distracting visuals or inadequate visuals. Demonstrates little creativity.	No more than two errors in spelling, word usage, or punctuation. Font size and/or selection appropriate on some slides. Good use of color and contrast. Demonstrates only moderate creativity.	No errors in spelling, word usage, or punctuation. Font size and/or selection appropriate. Good use of color and contrast. Appropriate use of visuals. Demonstrates exemplary creativity.
Use of active teaching strategies and audience involvement (10)	Speaker reads or speaks continuously with no active learning strategies or audience involvement.	Minimal audience involvement or use of active learning strategies.	Effective use of active learning strategies and audience involvement.	Exemplary use of active learning strategies and audience involvement with methods such as questioning, clickers and/or poll questions, and/or case studies.

Total points possible: 100   **Score and summary comments:**

CONCLUSION

Presentations allow students the opportunity to share their work with their student peers. A presentation also allows the educator an opportunity to evaluate the students' knowledge of the selected or assigned topic, their ability to find and evaluate professional references related to the topic, their project-planning skills, and their communication skills. With a well-designed assignment description that includes the scoring rubric, students are motivated and prepared to succeed in presentation assignments.

8

Participation

The inclusion of participation in evaluation plans for college courses is controversial. There is a clear difference between attendance and participation. If participation is included in the evaluation plan for a course, that participation must relate to course objectives and be purposeful.

By the end of this chapter, you will learn how to:

- Describe reasons to use participation for evaluation
- Discuss methods to encourage participation
- Design a clear assignment description for participation for evaluation
- Identify prerequisite knowledge and/or resources required by students for participation
- Develop or adapt a scoring rubric for participation

USING PARTICIPATION FOR EVALUATION

Participation refers to the contribution of the student to class discussion and other class activities. Because evaluation methods must relate to course objectives, attendance alone is not participation and should not contribute to a student's summative evaluation and grade. However, while credit should not be granted for simply attending class, failure to attend class does result in loss of participation points since the student cannot participate if he or she is not present.

Croxall (2010) writes what many of us believe; the reason to grade students' participation is so that students will come prepared. Since teaching is a lot more difficult when students are not ready to interact on the course content and objectives, he views participation as the carrot that aids in student engagement. Educators want students to learn from one another.

When discussion and questioning is added to the passive teaching strategy of lecture, learning becomes more active. If students know that the expectation is that they participate in the discussion and volunteer answers to questions posed, they are more likely to be involved in the active learning process. Discussion encourages students in the development of language and public speaking skills, as well as social interaction with sharing of ideas. Active learning strategies such as class discussion increases what is remembered and facilitates application, analysis, evaluation, and synthesis.

In a study by Kraus and Sears (2008) investigating student and teacher perceptions of selected pedagogical techniques, students perceived discussion of particular value and identified telling of personal stories as an effective learning tool. Both discussion and shared stories contribute to building a sense of community.

The Teaching Center at Washington University at Saint Louis (2009) describes various types of participants. Extraverts typically think while they speak and are the preeminent active learner and participant. Introverts are typically reflective learners who typically develop ideas in their minds before speaking; they are likely to be initially quiet as they formulate their thoughts. Other students may be shy and hesitant to speak, especially if they must compete with the more vocal students.

When participation is used for summative evaluation and contributes to the student's grade, the learning environment must provide varied opportunities for participation, the ability for all students to participate, and a reasonable way to evaluate the level of contribution. Varying opportunities for participation, such as discussion or group projects, will allow students to participate when the topics or learning activities are those where they are most likely to excel. Efforts must be made to allow all students to participate and prevent the monopolization of the discussion by one or more very vocal students. One method described by Bean and Peterson (1998) was to use 3×5 index cards with the name of one student on each card. These cards were shuffled and then one selected and the student whose name was on that card was questioned. His or her response was then rated by the educator and marked on the card. This method would certainly help with the issue of remembering whether a student was an active participant in discussion and the quality of the student's response. Students were informed that this technique would be used and the expectations for responses. While this method would certainly encourage participation, as supported by a more recent study by Dallimore, Hertenstein, and Platt (2004) using this same cold-calling strategy, it would also likely increase anxiety for adult learners.

Finally, it is not reasonable for an educator to expect to be able to objectively evaluate an individual student's contribution with very large class sizes. Even in smaller classes, it is a good idea to keep notes regarding students' participation immediately after class. Maznevski (1996) recommends that the educator sit down with the class list with photographs and rate each student's contribution for that day from 0 to 4 (Table 8.1). Another advantage to this method is that it becomes obvious to the educator that he or she is consistently failing to engage a specific student and efforts can be made during successive class sessions to encourage the student's participation.

Challenges and Criticism to Using Participation in Student Evaluation

Though most evaluation plans do include a student's participation in the final grade for a course (Croxall, 2010; Weimer, 2011), use of participation for summative evaluation certainly has opponents. The major issues include subjectivity and resultant grade challenges, penalization of quiet and/or shy students, and inadequate feedback for improvement.

Many consider assessment of student participation to be too subjective, which may contribute to grade challenges and discourse with students. Students are most likely to challenge participation grades

TABLE 8.1   Class Participation Summary Score for Each Class Session

Score	Description
0	• Absent, disruptive, disrespectful, or frequent efforts to monopolize conversation
1	• Not disruptive or disrespectful • Responds only when called on but responses offer no evidence of preparation
2	• Occasional spontaneous response and responses show evidence of preparation • Responses are primarily a reiteration of assigned readings or viewings but no evidence of application or analysis
3	• Frequent spontaneous involvement in discussion • Responses show evidence of application and analysis
4	• Frequent spontaneous involvement in discussion • Responses show evidence of synthesis and evaluation • Responds thoughtfully to other students' responses • Suggests divergent approaches to facilitate understanding

Adapted from Maznevski (1996).

because they perceive them to be subjective and, possibly, capricious. They are more likely to argue about their participation grade than a midterm examination. Anecdotal notes and recording a score with each class session will help you remember why you awarded the grade that you did. One strategy is to record full participation points in the grade book at the beginning of the term and then deduct as necessary. Students will likely come to you and ask the reason for the deduction, which will allow you to give constructive feedback for improvement. Feedback related to the quality of participation being rarely given is another concern regarding participation grades. Multhaup (2008) recommends providing feedback several times during the term.

Another valid concern is that quiet, less vocal students are at a disadvantage when participation is a part of the evaluation plan (Davis, 1993), though they may be very strong students who complete their preparation for class and do well on papers and examinations. English as a second language (ESL) students, students with disabilities, and minority students are likely to be included in the group of less vocal students who are likely to be awarded fewer participation points. Another issue to consider is that students may say anything that comes into their head so that they get those participation points rather than think about the subject and contribute value to the conversation.

Evaluation of participation is exceptionally valuable in the "flipped classroom," where students are expected to use learning materials developed and/or selected by the educator prior to coming to class (Critz & Knight, 2013). The student is then expected to participate in active learning strategies such as discussion, case studies, or problem-based learning. It is important to objectively evaluate the student's preparation and participation with this pedagogical approach.

Facilitation of Participation

A consideration in ensuring an opportunity for all students to participate is the layout of the room. A room with movable chairs will facilitate discussion much better than an auditorium. Moving chairs into a circle or a U so that students can see and speak to one another will also encourage discussion (The Teaching Center at Washington University, 2009). Using name tents so that you perceive students as individuals and student peers can address one another by name is useful (The Teaching Center at Washington University, 2009).

Some techniques that the educator may use that will encourage and focus discussion include:

- Clarify expectations
- Set ground rules
- Arrange the physical space
- Use verbal and nonverbal cues
- Allow time for thought before response; tolerate silences
- Avoid interrupting students and discourage interruption by other students
- Vary your reinforcement and encouraging comments; avoid value statements such as "good answer" since failure to say the same in another instance may imply that it was not a good answer

- Summarize and/or clarify student responses
- Limit your own comments; again, tolerate silences
- Keep the discussion on track
- Encourage quiet students
- Avoid allowing a student to monopolize the conversation
- Emphasize a student's comment by referring back to the comment when appropriate
- Summarize when needed (The Teaching Center at Washington University, 2009; deYoung, 2008).

While most agree that it is reasonable to make participation, and indirectly class preparation, a portion of the evaluation plan for a course, it should not be a large portion of the final course grade. In most nursing courses, it is very difficult to justify more than 5% to 10% of the grade being based on preparation and participation.

WRITING THE ASSIGNMENT DESCRIPTION

Start your assignment description by linking preparation and active participation to active learning. Clearly explain the participation expectations such as volunteering answers to questions posed, providing respectful responses to discussion questions and opinions of their fellow students, and being a productive member during group activities. Explain that just saying "something" does not warrant a positive evaluation of participation but rather that any response must be thoughtful and respectful. It is important to stress that the quality of the contribution is more significant than the quantity of contribution, lest there be encouragement of irrelevant vocalizations. If you have an expectation that students do contribute to discussion with every class session, indicate that. However, it is more likely that you would want the student to speak up when he or she has a thoughtful answer or opinion rather than just speaking to get those "points" during each session. Also, indicate that only respectful discourse is acceptable.

You should include strategies that might be used during class to facilitate effective discussion and universal participation. Explain that students who do not raise their hand or volunteer comments may be called on and that students who are frequent contributors may be asked to temporarily withhold response to allow other students to participate.

Consider involving the students in clarifying expectations and ground rules for participation. Multhaup (2008) suggests group discussion of the following questions.

- What kind of contributions in class are worth listening to or, if on discussion board, worth reading?
- What kind of contributions are helpful for learning course content/concepts?
- What kind of contributions are not helpful?

It is important to inform students that flattering the professor or degrading other students will not result in a better participation score. Rather, the contribution of the student to the learning and understanding of others is the greatest value.

IDENTIFYING PRIOR KNOWLEDGE AND/OR RESOURCES TO BE AVAILABLE FOR STUDENTS

Clear communication regarding learning activities required prior to each class session is vital. Students are expected to have completed this preparatory work and failure to do so is frequently obvious. If the student does say something that is not consistent with the readings, you can ask for the basis of their response or opinion.

Communication skills, either verbal or written, are required for clear and succinct delivery of thoughts and opinions. Participation in class or in a synchronous classroom using Adobe Connect or Blackboard Illuminate requires students to not only formulate their thoughts and opinions but to do so with respect to others' thoughts and opinions.

MODIFYING FOR ONLINE DELIVERY

If you are using synchronous sessions using videoconferencing, audioconferencing, or chat room, discussion is as it is in the classroom. You should ask the student to identify him- or herself if there is not a distinct way to determine identity through the methods being used. If you are using videoconferencing including software platforms such as Adobe Connect or Blackboard Illuminate, the student also has the option to type in the chat box rather than speak out. Many students are more comfortable doing this. Also, be clear about whether students need to click on the "raise hand" button rather than speaking out.

If you are using asynchronous delivery only, participation is likely through a threaded discussion board process. Chapter 9 describes the use of discussion board for evaluation.

EVALUATING PARTICIPATION

As discussed earlier, evaluating participation can be a challenge, especially with large classes. It is important to keep anecdotal notes throughout the term to help substantiate the scores that you award for participation. The following scoring rubric (Table 8.2) can be adapted to include your specific expectations for student participation.

Peer Participation in Evaluation

Melvin (1988) described a process where students used a three-point scale for evaluation of participation of student peers at the end of the semester. A 3 would correlate to a C, a 2 would correlate to a B, and a 1 would correlate to an A. These peer ratings were only used if significantly higher than the educator's grade. Since the peer evaluation could only benefit and could not penalize, students were more accepting of the process.

TABLE 8.2 Modifiable Grading Rubric for Participation

Criteria (Points Possible)	Does Not Meet Expectations	Nearly Meets Expectations	Meets Expectations	Exceeds Expectations	Score and Comments
Evidence of preparation for class (25)	< 18	18–20	21–23	24–25	
	• Frequently no evidence of preparation	• Usually demonstrates evidence of preparation	• Consistently demonstrates evidence of preparation	• Consistently demonstrates evidence of exceptional preparation by reading beyond required readings	
Demonstration of knowledge/ reasoning during class	< 18	18–20	21–23	24–25	
	• Lack of knowledge impairs ability to reason • Frequently expresses opinion without grounds	• Some knowledge gaps limit ability to reason • Occasionally expresses opinions without grounds	• Synthesis of core knowledge with ability to make and defend a scholarly argument • Rarely expresses opinions without grounds	• Superior synthesis of core knowledge with ability to make and defend a scholarly argument • Never expresses opinions without grounds	
Contribution during class session (25)	< 18	18–20	21–23	24–25	
	• Silent most of the time	• Minimal contribution or dominates the conversation or unable to communicate clearly	• Regular participation without dominating the conversation • Communicates clearly • Occasionally engages other students with ideas, questions, and constructive feedback	• Regular and exceptional participation with provision of insight and thoughts that advance the discussion • Communicates effectively • Consistently engages other students with ideas, questions, and constructive feedback	

(continued)

TABLE 8.2 Modifiable Grading Rubric for Participation (*continued*)

Criteria (Points Possible)	Does Not Meet Expectations	Nearly Meets Expectations	Meets Expectations	Exceeds Expectations	Score and Comments
	< 18	18–20	21–23	24–25	
Demonstration of respect, responsibility, accountability, and leadership during class (25)	• Frequently late for class • Rude, disruptive, dominating, and/or inconsiderate/ disrespectful of others	• Frequently late • Frequently disruptive, dominating, and/or disrespectful of others' opinions • Inattentive listener • Marginally participative team member	• Rarely late • Usually caring, respectful, and encouraging to others • Usually good listener • Actively listens • Excellent team member and occasionally serves as a leader while encouraging and appreciating the contributions of others	• Always on time • Consistently caring, respectful, and encouraging of others • Consistently active listener • Excellent team member and consistently serves as a leader while encouraging and appreciating the contributions of others	

Total points possible: 100	Score and summary comments:

CONCLUSION

While using class preparation and participation in summative evaluation is controversial, it is very common and most college courses include participation in the evaluation plan. With the inclusion of participation in summative evaluation, efforts must be made to clearly communicate expectations to students and to design the learning environment to allow all students to participate.

9

Discussion Board

Nurse educators in online or blended courses frequently use discussion board threaded discussion as either a substitute or a supplement to course discussion in a face-to-face classroom. This chapter focuses on the evaluation of student participation through online discussion board assignments. The use of discussion board assignments as a teaching/learning strategy and evaluation method is explored. Lastly, this chapter presents the five phases of discussion board assignment design and development.

By the end of this chapter, you will learn how to:

- Describe reasons for the use of a discussion board for evaluation
- Design a clear assignment description for threaded discussion through a discussion board for evaluation
- Identify prerequisite knowledge and/or resources required by students for effective use of a discussion board for evaluation
- Develop or adapt a scoring rubric for a discussion board assignment

USING DISCUSSION BOARDS FOR EVALUATION

In online asynchronous course content delivery, class communication and student participation methods vary widely. Most teaching and learning takes place through computer-mediated technologies such as the course learning management system and discussion board. In this online environment, "students must attain their learning of course content and processes from required readings, materials such as slide presentations on course websites (e.g., using software such as PowerPoint or Echo360), content available through the Internet, and a variety of assignments" (Lunney & Sammarco, 2009, p. 26).

As an active learning strategy, students often communicate with each other and the educator via discussion board by answering a series of educator-guided questions related to the assigned course material, and discussing those answers through threaded discussions with other students (Bender, 2012). Baglione and Nastanski (2007) indicate that discussion boards supplement content delivery by allowing students to be active participants through discourse with other students and educators. Nurse educators, as an extension to their delivery of new content, post questions related to the content students will respond to via discussion board. Students will respond to each other's original postings, provide substantive comments, post new questions, and debate details. Educators will also post to select discussions to provide clarity, correct misconceptions, refocus the conversation, or present an alternative perspective students have overlooked. It is through these threaded student postings on the discussion board that educators evaluate student participation (Bender, 2012).

WRITING THE ASSIGNMENT DESCRIPTION

Writing a discussion board assignment typically requires the educator to work through five phases of design and development (Figure 9.1). Steps for developing each phase of a discussion board assignment are outlined below.

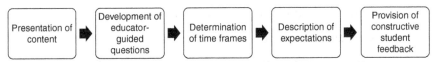

FIGURE 9.1 Five phases of design and development of a discussion board assignment.

Present Content

- Determine what content will be included in each learning module.
- Determine how that content will be presented to the student. Content can be presented through myriad ways including required readings, PowerPoint, Echo360, Camtasia, other types of presentation software, and Internet resources.

Develop Educator-Guided Questions Related To Content

- Based on the content presented, create questions that encourage students to think critically, provide well-supported opinions, engage in discussion, and participate in lively debate.
- Avoid asking a question that requires the student to simply regurgitate facts. It will only serve to limit meaningful discussion and class participation.

Describe the Expectations for Participation

- Determine the expected frequency of contributions.
  - Be clear about expectations of the primary post.
  - Determine frequency and expectations for secondary posts (i.e., response to another student or educator's post).

Determine Time Frames for Each Assignment Segment

- Remind students that all posts should be timely. Encourage students to begin posting well before the assignment completion date.

- Identify due dates for the following assignment phases:
  - Review of content
  - Student's original post response to the educator-guided, content-related questions
  - Student's response(s) to the original and subsequent posts of other students and educators
  - Discussion board assignment completion date
- Determine how substantive each student's post should be. In each response (post), consider the student's:
  - Accuracy of the response
  - Thoughtfulness, insight, and analysis
  - Ability to connect prior learned content, content learned outside of class, and real-life experience
  - Contribution to the learning of others
  - Strategic use of references
  - Use of grammar, professionally appropriate vocabulary, and correct spelling

Provide Feedback

- Provide ample, substantive, and regular feedback on the student's participation and contribution to the course.
- Use a scoring rubric (see sample scoring rubric at the end of this chapter).
- Consider asking students to perform a self-evaluation of their participation at regular intervals throughout the course.

PRIOR KNOWLEDGE AND/OR RESOURCES TO BE AVAILABLE TO STUDENTS

Students should have a strong understanding of the expectations related to online courses. You may consider developing an online discussion orientation so students can gain the technical information necessary to participate in productive conversations (Bender, 2012). Familiarity with the learning management system or discussion board software is essential. Students will also require resources on American Psychological Association (APA) style for their references. If you do not require they buy the APA manual, you may consider providing the URL to Owl Purdue Online Writing Lab (owl.english .purdue.edu/owl/resource/560/01) in the assignment description.

EVALUATING THE DISCUSSION BOARD ASSIGNMENT

Use the following modifiable rubric (Table 9.1) for discussion board assignments to evaluate students in the following categories: frequency of contributions, accuracy of facts and evidence of critical thinking, sources, voice, and grammar and spelling.

TABLE 9.1 Modifiable Scoring Rubric for Discussion Board Assignment

Category (Points Possible)	Poor	Fair	Good	Excellent	Score and Comments
Met expectation for frequency of contributions (10)	**0** The student did not post at all.	**8** Student participated in ___ primary posts and ___ secondary responses	**9** Student participated in ___ primary posts and ___ secondary responses	**10** Student participated in ___ primary posts and ___ secondary responses	
Accuracy of facts and evidence of critical thinking (30)	**≤21** No referenced facts are reported or are inaccurately reported. Response contains misinformation and/or inaccurate thinking related to the case.	**22–24** Most referenced facts are reported accurately. Response demonstrates limited knowledge of content and no critical thinking related to the case.	**25–27** Almost all referenced facts are reported accurately. Response shows knowledge of content but limited critical thinking related to the case.	**28–30** All referenced facts are reported accurately. Response shows substantive knowledge of content and demonstrates significant critical thinking related to the question or case.	
Sources (20)	**≤14** Based solely on personal opinion or lay literature. Multiple errors in APA citations and references.	**15–16** References limited to textbooks or commercial (e.g., .com) websites. Several errors in APA citations and references.	**17–18** Multiple references including material from professional journals and noncommercial (e.g., .gov, .edu, .org) websites. Only one or two minor errors in APA citations or references.	**19–20** Multiple references including material from professional journals and noncommercial (e.g., .gov, .edu, .org) websites. At least one research article included in references. No errors in APA citations or references.	

	≤14	15–16	17–18	19–20
Voice (20)	The writer has not tried to transform the information in a personal way. The ideas and the way they are expressed seem to belong to someone else.	The writer relates some of his or her own knowledge or experience, but it adds nothing to the discussion of the topic.	The writer seems to be drawing on knowledge or experience, but there is some lack of ownership of the topic.	The writer seems to be writing from knowledge or experience. The author has taken the ideas and made them "his or her own."
	≤14	**15–16**	**17–18**	**19–20**
Grammar and spelling (20)	The writer makes more than four errors in spelling, word usage, sentence structure, grammar, or punctuation that distract the reader from the content.	The writer makes three or four errors in spelling, word usage, sentence structure, grammar, or punctuation that distract the reader from the content.	The writer makes one or two errors in spelling, word usage, sentence structure, grammar, or punctuation that distract the reader from the content.	The writer makes no errors in spelling, word usage, sentence structure, grammar, or punctuation that distract the reader from the content.

Total points possible: 100   **Score and summary comments:**

CONCLUSION

Nurse educators in online or blended courses frequently use discussion board-threaded discussion as either a substitute or a supplement to course discussion in a face-to-face classroom. As an active learning strategy, students and educators can communicate with each other via discussion board by answering a series of educator-guided questions and discussion of those responses with each other. It is through these threaded communication postings that educators may evaluate student participation.

In order to effectively utilize the discussion board as a method of student evaluation, the educator must write a clear and comprehensive assignment description. The five phases of assignment description include: present content, develop educator-guided questions related to content, describe the expectations for participation, determine time frames for each assignment segment, and provide meaningful and substantive feedback. Educators may use the modifiable scoring rubric for discussion board assignments in Table 9.1.

Reflective Journals

Educators frequently use reflective journals as a teaching/ learning strategy and a method of formative and summative evaluation with students in undergraduate and graduate settings (Oermann & Gaberson, 2014). They may be used as an assignment in didactic or clinical courses to enhance translation of content into real-world experiences and facilitate critical-thinking skills (Iwaoka & Crosetti, 2007; Langley & Brown, 2010). Reflective journals are one of the few assignments that support affective learning and promote the development of life-long, self-directed learning.

By the end of this chapter, you will learn how to:

- Describe reasons to use reflective journaling for evaluation
- Design a clear assignment description for a reflective journal assignment for evaluation
- Identify prerequisite knowledge and/or resources required by students for quality reflective journals
- Guide students using various media for reflective journals
- Develop or adapt a scoring rubric for evaluation of reflective journals

USING REFLECTIVE JOURNALS FOR EVALUATION

A reflective journal is an assignment and evaluation method that facilitates student connection of didactic knowledge with their real world (Oermann & Gaberson, 2014). The purpose of a reflective journal is to stimulate deep learning and critical self-reflection and analysis for personal and professional growth (Iwaoka & Crosetti, 2007). The process of reflective journaling provides the learning connection between the cognitive, psychomotor, and affective learning domains for the student (Bolin, Khramtsova, & Saamio, 2005). Cognitive learning is enhanced through guided reflections by the educator, which facilitate the student's linking of the theory to the life experience. Affective learning is supported as reflective journaling promotes student inquiry and understanding of the value, relevance, and moral and ethical implications of the content being learned through experience (Bolin et al., 2005). Reflective journaling as a teaching method supports the students' owning their learning experience and their ultimate responsibility for their own learning.

Reflective journaling requires that the student know the course content and expectations. The student must also have self-awareness and confidence to explore factors that impacted their learning process before, during, and after the learning experience. It moves the student beyond the basic recollection of theoretical, classroom facts into practical application. Self-reflection and journaling can be intimidating to students as it forces them to look at what they are doing, whether or not it worked, their own strengths and weaknesses, and to explore knowledge gaps related to a particular situation where they may have needed to use a different or more effective approach (Hong & Chew, 2008). As a goal of this assignment is to facilitate student self-motivation, empowerment, and growth, the process and structure for the reflective journal must be clear and presented in a manner that is helpful and safe for the student.

Educators can use reflective journaling as a classroom assignment to facilitate student understanding of how content and concepts taught can be applied and integrated into their own life experience or understanding (Hubert, 2010). In simulation and clinical situations, reflective journaling enables the student to look at expectations and preparation of the learning experience, the actual events of the learning experience, their response to the learning experience, and exploration of factors that might have enhanced the learning experience. As an assignment, reflective journaling provides a model and process for the student to become a life-long learner, with self-awareness and confidence.

Additional types of reflective journals identified in educational literature include dialogue journals and reflective class or team journals. Dialogue journals are kept jointly by the learner and the educator. Often the learner is answering questions presented by the educator about a specific area of interest. The educator continues questioning through feedback to facilitate the learner's exploration and elaboration (Linnell, 2010). A class or team may also share reflective journals collectively to openly communicate and share ideas. In these types of journals, the educator often models reflections and challenges the learners to increase the depth complexity of their inquiries and observations (Hubert, 2010). Thus it is important that the educator be clear on the type of journal assigned and how this will be evaluated.

Experiential learning models, which emphasize learning as an active process that involves reflection, support the use of reflective journaling. Building on this, Gibbs (1988) developed a model for reflection to support learning that includes the following six stages: description, feelings, evaluation, analysis, conclusions, and action plan. These stages provide the student with a foundation and process for reflective journaling. The stages of the reflective cycle, and examples of questions to guide reflective journaling, are presented in Table 10.1.

TABLE 10.1 Questions to Guide Reflective Journaling

Stage	Focus	Guiding Questions
Description	Describe the experience as clearly, factually, and succinctly as possible.	Where were you? Who was there? What happened? What did you do? What were others doing?
Feelings	Describe your thoughts and feelings before, during, and after the experience.	What did you think before, during, and after the experience? How did you feel before, during, and after the experience?

(continued)

TABLE 10.1   Questions to Guide Reflective Journaling (*continued*)

Stage	Focus	Guiding Questions
Evaluation	Describe the outcome of the experience and your contribution to the outcome.	How well did you do in or with this experience? What went well? What could have gone better? Was this a good or bad experience? What were your strengths/weaknesses in this experience?
Analysis	Identify the factors that influenced the success or challenges in the experience.	What helped you in this experience? What might have helped you in this experience? What hindered you in this experience? How does what you have learned from lectures, readings, and other experiences relate or compare with this experience?
Conclusions	Describe what you learned from this experience and how this learning can be applied in the future.	What would you do the same? What would you do differently? How has this experience changed you? How might what you learned be applied in the future?
Action plan	Describe a plan for additional learning and/or skill development identified through the experience.	What can you take from this experience to use in the future? What will you do differently as a result of this experience? What specific action is needed to better apply what was learned? How will you obtain the knowledge or skills to perform better in similar situations?

Adapted from Gibbs (1998).

WRITING THE ASSIGNMENT DESCRIPTION

Clearly identify the purpose of the reflective journal and the student-learning objectives being addressed. Provide an explanation of what a reflective journal is, and review the required elements of the reflective journal with the students. Provide the rubric that will be used to grade the reflective journal to the students at the outset and address any questions. It is important that the students realize that the focus of the reflective journal is on them and their learning process. Direct the students to select an experience to reflect on. A simple structure that incorporates the required elements for the reflection (Table 10.1) helps guide the students' reflection. It is helpful to emphasize that a reflective journal is not a diary. The format for reflective journaling is most often written. It can be completed electronically or with paper and pencil. If students hand-write their journals, remind them that illegible journals will not count or be graded. For a reflective journal that the student may be transporting on a regular basis, such as a clinical journal, a simple, flat, three-ring paper folder where all of the journal pages can be secured is recommended. This avoids students using large binders that can be unwieldy to transport and papers flying if folders are dropped. Students should keep all the journal entries together, in chronological order, labeling them accordingly. This is helpful when giving formative feedback, tracking the students' responses, and evaluating their growth and learning over time. Often a sample of well-written reflection is helpful in getting students started with the reflective process. An example of a written reflective journal entry is provided in Table 10.2.

TABLE 10.2 Sample of Reflective Journaling

Description	Today I provided care for a 79-year-old man with Alzheimer's disease (AD), who had been admitted for an abrupt change in mental status and level of consciousness and tachycardia. I talked with him, assisted him with his bath and meals, ambulated and monitored his orientation, level of consciousness, and vital signs. I needed help with understanding the monitors and by the end of the day could keep an eye on the monitor and the patient at the same time.
Feelings	Today was my first day on the telemetry unit. I was worried about taking care of a cardiac patient being monitored and really felt overwhelmed when I realized that he also had AD. This was a totally new experience for me and I was afraid that I would miss a critical piece of information or do something wrong and harm the patient. The patient kept repeating things over and over and asking the same questions. This was frustrating but I was patient with him and addressed his questions. This patient reminded me a lot of my grandfather who passed away several years ago, which made me feel sad but I really wanted to do a good job taking care of him. Because of his confusion, I wasn't sure what I could believe or not of what he said. This added to the worry that I would miss something important. I felt I did the best I could do today but I was exhausted at the end of the day.

(continued)

TABLE 10.2   Sample of Reflective Journaling (*continued*)

Evaluation	Initially I was overwhelmed taking care of this complex patient. I think I did a good job taking care of this patient today. Initially I was overwhelmed by how his AD would complicate the care. I knew that I needed to be very observant for any changes in his mental or cardiac status and that he may not be able to tell me about any problems that he was having. My patience and ability to provide care to him was a definite strength. I safely monitored the patient and became familiar with the leads and monitors. I still need to get more comfortable taking care of patients with complex needs.
Analysis	Initially I was overwhelmed with the monitors and dealing with the patient; however, as I got used to them I was able to use them to monitor the patient just as we had reviewed in class. While I learned about AD last semester, I realized that I probably haven't retained as much as I needed to and I will need to review that information. Because the patient reminded me of my grandfather, I found myself responding to him and helping him like I always did with my grandfather. More information about the patient's baseline cognitive status would have been helpful in working with this patient. I did a lot for the patient and should probably have tried to see what he could do for himself.
Conclusions/ learning	Working with patients who have dementia certainly adds a whole new level of complexity to the plan of care in the telemetry setting. You have to rely on your observations and look for subtle changes in behavior that the patient may not be able to directly verbalize. His cardiac status remained stable throughout the shift with only small variations in rhythm with activity. It would've been helpful to know more about his baseline so that I could encourage his functioning at that level and not do too much for him, as well as be sure I wasn't expecting too much. This is information that I would actively want to seek out, perhaps from the patient's family or from others who know him best. It would also be helpful to have a reference book close by of simple activities that can be used with this type of patient to keep him occupied and engaged. Given that the population is aging it is likely that I will see more and more patients who have dementia in acute medical settings. This may be an area that I could specialize in.
Action plan	Review information on dementia and how that may affect patient care. Develop a list of simple activities that can be easily done with patients who have dementia. Review information from lecture on taking care of patients in the telemetry unit.

MODIFYING FOR ONLINE DELIVERY

Students may submit electronic journals to a designated drop box using your institution's learning management system or other software. It is helpful to have the journal set up in a sequential manner so that previous entries can be easily viewed. For clarity, have a consistent format for the title so that it is easy to find each journal entry. Consider student's last name, first initial, journal entry number, and date as required elements for the online entry (e.g., SMITHA1d-dmmyy). Thus, if needed, the journal entries can be easily printed in consecutive order. Another option is having the student set up the journal as a collaborative document on a platform such as Google Docs. This provides the opportunity for the instructor to respond to the student in a dialogue. Instruct the student to add new entries at the top of the document to prevent having to scroll through all old entries to get to the new entry.

Audio and video recordings can also be a useful medium for students to document their reflective journaling (Parikh, Janson, & Singleton, 2012). This method of reflective journaling requires that the student have access to video or audio recording equipment and that the educator have the means to download and access the recordings. The benefit of an audio or video reflective journal is that they capture the nuances of voice and nonverbal communication that convey so much but are often missing in text.

EVALUATING THE REFLECTIVE JOURNAL

Decide and clearly communicate to the students how the reflective journal will be graded. Some educators will assign a grade to each journal entry. Particularly when students are new to reflective journaling, this process can be quite intimidating and summative grading of the initial reflective journal entries may undermine the formative evaluation process. Other educators support the reflective journaling process in a formative manner, emphasizing that by the end of a designated period of time (i.e., mid-way through the course or perhaps by the end of the course), the reflection(s) in the journal should be developed more completely and meet the identified expectations with the expected depth. Initial entries are often more superficial and lack the depth that comes with ongoing experience. Provide feedback to the student as quickly as possible on how to effectively reflect and journal. Emphasizing that this is a process that will improve over time often relieves student anxiety about the reflective journaling process. It is important to note that the student's reflections are private and should not be shared by the instructor without the student's consent. The student needs to know that his or her journal entries are confidential. This provides the students the freedom to deal with their experiences openly and honestly without fear of embarrassment or retaliation. The following scoring rubric can be modified for use in evaluation of a reflective journal assignment (Table 10.3)

CONCLUSION

A reflective journal is an assignment and evaluation method that provides students an opportunity to connect didactic knowledge with their real-world experience through application of that knowledge by written or verbal means. It is a viable alternative to testing by examination and provides an opportunity for students to demonstrate achievement of higher-level student-learning objectives in cognitive and affective learning domains. A well-designed scoring rubric provides a consistent method for collecting data regarding the student's level of achievement of learning objective. These data can be used in formative and summative evaluation processes.

TABLE 10.3 Modifiable Rubric for a Reflective Journal

Criterion (Points Possible)	Does Not Meet Expectations	Nearly Meets Expectations	Meets Expectations	Exceeds Expectations	Score and Comments
	≤ 7	8	9	10	
Description of the experience (10)	Journal provides description of the learning experience as vague or disorganized or a significant aspect of the learning experience is not clearly identified.	Journal provides a description of the learning experience with a few gaps in detail that impact clarity; at least one significant aspect of the experience is identified.	Journal provides adequate description of the learning experience and identifies and describes significant aspects of the experience in a clear, organized, logical manner.	Journal provides a detailed description of the learning experience in a clear, succinct, organized, and logical manner and identifies and describes significant aspects of the learning.	
	≤ 7	8	9	10	
Description of thoughts and feelings (10)	Journal superficially describes a thought or feeling associated with specific aspects of the learning experience.	Journal describes a thought and feeling associated with specific aspects of the learning experience.	Journal describes several positive and negative thoughts and feelings and how they persist or change throughout the learning experience.	Journal describes a full range (i.e., positive and negative) of thoughts and feelings and how they persist or change throughout the learning experience.	

(continued)

TABLE 10.3 Modifiable Rubric for a Reflective Journal (*continued*)

Criterion (Points Possible)	Does Not Meet Expectations	Nearly Meets Expectations	Meets Expectations	Exceeds Expectations	Score and Comments
	≤ 14	15–16	17–18	19–20	
Evaluation (20)	Journal identifies how well the experience went but with minimal connection with thoughts or feelings to the overall experience, or fails to include identification of own strength or weakness in the experience.	Journal identifies how well the experience went, incorporating the impact of thoughts or feelings and identification of own strength and weakness impacting the experience.	Journal includes discussion of how well the experience went, incorporating the ongoing impact of thoughts and feelings and discussion of own strengths and weaknesses and how they impacted the overall experience.	Journal includes exploration of how well the experience went, incorporating the ongoing impact of various thoughts and feelings identified, making specific connections to the overall experience, and includes a detailed discussion of own strengths and weaknesses and how they impacted the experience.	

	≤14	15–16	17–18	19–20
Analysis (20)	Journal includes minimal self-reflection.	Journal includes self-reflection and discussion of at least one possible rationale for why the experience went the way it did.	Journal includes self-reflection and discussion of possible rationales for why the experience went the way it did; includes discussion of several factors (i.e., positive and negative) that may have contributed to the experience; journal includes limited discussion of other possible interpretations.	Journal includes self-reflection and discussion of possible rationales for why the experience went the way it did; includes thorough exploration of a wide variety of factors (i.e., positive and negative) that may have contributed to the experience; journal includes exploration of other possible interpretations.
Conclusions/ learning (20)	Learning is not clearly identified or discussed and there is failure to identify how learning can be applied in future situations.	Learning and application to a future situation is clearly identified with minimal discussion.	Learning and application to future situations is clearly identified and discussed.	Learning and application to a variety of future situations is clearly and thoroughly identified and discussed.

(continued)

TABLE 10.3 Modifiable Rubric for a Reflective Journal (*continued*)

Criterion (Points Possible)	Does Not Meet Expectations	Nearly Meets Expectations	Meets Expectations	Exceeds Expectations	Score and Comments
	≤ 10	11–12	13–14	15	
Action plan (15)	Action plan identified is broad and nonspecific.	Journal identifies a specific action to be taken to support learning but no time frame identified.	Journal identifies specific action steps to be taken to support learning and identifies a timeline for completion.	Journal identifies specific actions to be taken to support learning and a detailed strategy for completion with specific resources identified.	
	< 3.5	3.5	4	5	
Legibility, grammar, and spelling (5)	Journal is illegible or includes many errors in spelling, word usage, sentence structure, grammar, or punctuation that distract the reader from the content.	Journal is legible with several errors in spelling, word usage, sentence structure, grammar, or punctuation that distract the reader from the content.	Journal is legible with only minor errors in spelling, word usage, sentence structure, grammar, or punctuation that do not distract the reader from the content.	Journal is legible with no errors in spelling, word usage, sentence structure, grammar, or punctuation that distract the reader from the content.	
Total points possible: 100	**Score and summary comments:**				

11

Case Studies

The use of case studies as an effective teaching and learning strategy and method of evaluation is popular across many academic disciplines including nursing, medicine, law, business, and the social sciences (Popil, 2011). In nursing, educators utilize case studies to provide students with real-life or imagined clinical patient experiences, without risking the safety of real patients. Case studies are a "method of storytelling that gives students access to the human experience and enables them to relate book learning to actual or invented human encounters" (Harrison, 2012, p. 67). Leenders et al. (as cited in Popil, 2011, p. 205) defines a case study as a "description of an actual situation, commonly involving a decision, a challenge, and opportunity, a problem or an issue face by a person or persons in an organization." Case studies may also be referred to as case histories and case methods.

By the end of this chapter, you will learn how to:

- Describe reasons to use case studies for evaluation
- Appreciate advantages and challenges to using case studies for student evaluation

- Distinguish the most common types of case studies

- Create a case study

- Design a clear assignment description for presentations for evaluation

- Identify prerequisite knowledge and/or resources required by students for a presentation assignment

- Develop or adapt a scoring rubric for a presentation assignment

USING CASE STUDIES FOR EVALUATION

Popil (2011) contends that case studies should be based upon real-life or potential experiences; provide supporting data and documents to be analyzed, interpreted, and evaluated; and provide open-ended questions or problems for students to solve. The utilization of case study assignments is an effective supplement to traditional class-room presentations, and ensures that students can be active learners without fear of doing patient harm. Students can work on case study assignments independently, or within small groups in and out of the classroom, under the guidance of educators. Case studies are effective for evaluation in the cognitive and affective learning domains.

Evidence suggests that case studies can enhance a student's clinical problem-solving, decision-making, and critical-thinking skills (Grossman, Krom, & O'Connor, 2010; Harrison, 2012; Popil, 2011; Sprang, 2010). The utilization of case study assignments in nursing curricula is effective because case studies:

- Engage students in critical inquiry and reflective decision making

- Build a sense of collegiality

- Encourage students to engage in clinical assessment, clinical reasoning, and diagnostic and intervention skills in a safe environment

- Encourage higher-order thinking (i.e., higher levels in Bloom's taxonomy)

- Provide models of how expert practitioners think about actual clinical dilemmas (Popil, 2011)
- Increase students' repertoire of strategies by showing them how to approach problems (Popil, 2011)
- Help students learn to identify issues and think professionally about practical problems
- Provide emotional preparation for difficult future real-life situations

Clinical Pearl

Case studies can be used to improve and evaluate the student's critical thinking, decision-making, and clinical-reasoning skills.

Challenges to utilizing case studies as a teaching/learning strategy and evaluation method include:

- The student must be motivated to work through the case, access appropriate resources, and sometimes work in a team.
- The educator must be committed to the role of facilitator when using case studies. Case studies are not the time for lecturing, sharing stories, and impatiently answering your own case study questions.
- Case study development and implementation take considerable time and require an abundance of preparation.

TYPES OF CASE STUDIES

Case study formats can be categorized into six major case study types. These case study types and a description for their application in nursing education are described in Table 11.1.

TABLE 11.1   Major Types of Case Studies

Type of Case Study	Description
Analysis or issues case	• Teaches students analysis-level skills. • Requires students to *analyze* a case study relevant to topics in nursing. • May be submitted as an assignment or discussed openly under the guidance of the educator.
Extensive and detailed analysis case	• Centers on decisions and interventions made by others, the patients affected by these decisions and interventions, and the impact of the decision on all stakeholders (e.g., patient, family, medical team, organization, community, etc.). • Requires the student to read the case and provide an analysis of the decision and interventions, and makes recommendations for change. • May be submitted as an assignment or discussed openly under the direction of the educator.
Dilemma or decision case	• Presents an individual patient, family, institution, or community faced with a problem that must be solved by the student(s). • Includes three distinct sections: (1) introduction of problem, (2) background to understand the situation, and (3) a narrative section that explains recent events leading up to the problem. • Requires the student to work through the information, analyze the problem(s), consider possible solutions and their likely consequences, and render a decision.
Directed case	• Includes short dramatic scenarios, accompanied by a list of "directed" questions that can be answered from lecture, textbook, and other familiar resources. • Poses questions that are typically closed-ended, with one correct answer (consider using multiple-choice response formats). • Requires students to work individually or in groups. • Provides an excellent choice for developing cases related to the care of the patient, especially in lower-level courses. • May be submitted as an assignment or presented to others in class.
Interrupted or unfolding case	• Presented to student(s) in segments in a progressive disclosure format. • Provides an excellent choice for developing cases that hone in on each of the multiple steps of caring for the patient. • Works well for students to work in groups and complete the case within a single class period, or as a take-home assignment where the student is presented the case in installments.

(continued)

TABLE 11.1   Major Types of Case Studies (*continued*)

Type of Case Study	Description
Problem-based learning (PBL)	• Requires students to work in small groups to find solutions to a presented problem(s), and works best in upper-level courses. • Involves students who work to identify the broad problem, identify what they know, and determine what they need to find out to develop a thoughtful and viable cogent solution. • Includes open-ended questions to narrow the focus and search for solutions. • Requires students to work through the problem(s) in the classroom, or as an outside assignment.

Source: National Center for Case Study Teaching in Science (2013).

CREATING A CASE STUDY

Before you can create a case study assignment, you must first develop a relevant case study. To create a clear and well-written case study, follow the development activities outlined in Table 11.2.

WRITING THE ASSIGNMENT DESCRIPTION

Once you create your case study and questions, you must now provide a clear and general description of your case study assignment. As with all assignment descriptions, it is imperative that you provide the student with a clear overview and purpose of the assignment. In the overview, connect the assignment to the relevant course and unit student-learning objectives. Next, describe the case study product. Will you require the student(s) to provide a verbal presentation of their findings and conclusions? Will you require students to answer the case study questions in writing? How will you evaluate your students?

Determining the due date will depend upon the case study student work product. If you require the student or group to present verbally prior to the end of class, those expectations should be clear in the instructions. If you assign the case study as a take-home, written assignment, include a due date and method for submission (e.g., e-mail,

TABLE 11.2   Guidelines for Developing a Well-Written Case Study

Development Activity	Description
Planning	• Identify course student-learning objective(s) this assignment is intended to evaluate. • Determine the intent of this student evaluation. Is it meant to be formative or summative? • Identify the purpose of the case study. What specifically are students expected to learn by completing the case study assignment? • Determine the setting. What is the environmental context in which the case study occurs? Depending on the type of case, there could be more than one relevant setting. • Determine the plot. Write a summary of events that will take place in the case. Answer the question, "What is supposed to happen in this case study?" • Determine the characters. Include only relevant characters in the case study. Examples include the patient and the patient's family, the nursing student, the nurse, the treatment team, etc. • Determine the pertinent information that will be included in the case study. Make certain it is appropriate for the student's current level of knowledge, and pertains to situations the students are most likely to encounter. • Be clear about what decisions and interventions you want your students to initiate (Gilboy & Kane, 2004). Anticipate the likely decisions and interventions your students will make.
Organizing	• Select an appropriate case study type (see Table 11.1). • Determine how and in what order the case study materials will be presented. Will you present the entire case study, or present segments of the case study in an unfolding or interrupted format?
Drafting	• Commit thoughts and ideas to paper. Write a rough draft. • Develop relevant questions related to the case. These questions should reflect the goals of the assignment and the unit and course student-learning objectives. Avoid writing fact-finding questions.
Revising	• Read and revise until you are comfortable with your work product. Be your own critical objective reader. • Ask a colleague to review the case, and revise as necessary. • Based on your experience and student feedback, revise after each time you present the case study.

Adapted from Lane (2007); Harrison (2012).

the assignment manager in the learning management system, your physical work mailbox, etc.). Remember, the more difficult the case study and the more complex the case study questions, the longer the student(s) will require to complete the assignment. Be clear about your expectations for early submissions, and the availability of feedback on draft papers.

Clearly state your expectations and parameters for answering the case study questions. Describe the appropriate response length. Expected response length can be anywhere between succinct short answers or well-referenced scholarly responses with no page limit. State your expectations for the use of American Psychological Association (APA) formatting and proper use of grammar. When appropriate, provide students a list of acceptable resources they can use when responding to the case study questions. If there are any off-limit resources (e.g., Wikipedia), list them accordingly. Lastly, explain the assignment rubric, and how the students can use that rubric as a guide for developing and submitting a quality product.

When developing a case study and case study assignment, consider these additional recommendations:

- Remember the case study is a supplement to other forms of learning. It is not an alternative. Typically, clinical case studies build upon previously learned knowledge. Examples of prior knowledge sources include traditional presentations and reading assignments. Providing students a case study they know nothing about, and have no prior knowledge from which to draw upon, will be a frustrating experience for both student and educator.

- If you plan to utilize a previously developed case study, adapt it to the needs of your current students, the unit and course learning objectives, and the appropriate level of cognitive ability (i.e., Bloom's taxonomy) you wish your students to achieve.

- Case studies and case study questions can be difficult and time-consuming to develop. Allow yourself enough time to create a quality assignment.

- The best case studies are as real-to-life as possible, are pertinent, and capture the students' full attention and participation (Gilboy & Kane, 2004).

If this is a group assignment, consider incorporating a peer evaluation so that you can determine if all students contributed to the final work product. Consider using the peer review included as Form 3.1.

PRIOR KNOWLEDGE AND/OR RESOURCES TO BE AVAILABLE TO STUDENTS

The success of case studies relies on the premise that students come to the case study with some level of prior knowledge. Students should be familiar with the topic through traditional teaching methods, assigned readings, and Internet and library searches. Students will also need to understand the basic fundamentals of case study assignments. Expect to provide guidance up front to avoid any significant misunderstandings. Depending upon assignment criteria, students may also be required to be proficient in APA for their references.

MODIFYING THE ASSIGNMENT FOR ONLINE USE

Students may verbally present their responses to the case study questions through the use of virtual classrooms such as Adobe Connect or Blackboard Illuminate. Depending upon the parameters of the assignment, students may be required to present using slides. Students who submit written responses may submit them via e-mail or through the assignment manager in the learning management system. Students may also respond to the case study questions in technological media such as discussion boards and collaborative documents (e.g., Google Docs and other Wikis).

EVALUATING THE CASE STUDY ASSIGNMENT

This section presents three types of case study scoring rubrics. Modifiable scoring rubric #1 (Table 11.3) should be used when you want to score the entire case study response section (i.e., all questions at once). Modifiable scoring rubric #2 (Table 11.4) is a simple, one-category assessment tool you can use to measure each individual case study question response. Modifiable scoring rubric #3 (Table 11.5) reflects a case study assignment that requires students to read a real-to-life case about a complex patient. Based on the information provided in the case study, students are asked to respond to a series of open-ended questions based on the nursing process. The rubric highlights the criteria necessary for successful student responses related to nursing process, and provides an opportunity for the educator to provide feedback on the quality of the case study responses in general.

CONCLUSION

The use of case studies as an effective teaching/learning strategy and method of evaluation is popular in nursing and other academic professions. In nursing, case studies provide students with a real life patient experience, without risking patient safety. Case studies can enhance the student's clinical problem-solving, decision-making, and critical-thinking skills. Case studies build a sense of collegiality, encourage higher-order thinking, provide models of how expert practitioners think about actual clinical dilemmas, and can even provide emotional preparation for difficult future real-life situations. Challenges to using case studies for student evaluation include student motivation, the educator's commitment to the role of facilitator, and the considerable time necessary to develop a case study.

Based upon the type of case study selected (Table 11.1), educators can create a case study that specifically meets the needs of the course. Steps in the development of case studies include planning, organizing, drafting, and revising. Next, the educator must write a clearly outlined assignment description. Lastly, the educator can use any of the modifiable case studies in Tables 11.3, 11.4, and 11.5.

TABLE 11.3 Modifiable Scoring Rubric #1 for a Case Study Assignment

Demonstration of Deeper Understanding and Cognitive Skills

Criterion	Does Not Meet Expectations	Nearly Meets Expectations	Meets Expectations	Exceeds Expectations	Score and Comments
				19–20	
Identification of the main issues/ problems	Unable to identify, label, and understand relevant main issues and/or problems	Identifies, labels, and understands all but 3 or 4 relevant main issues and/or problems	Identifies, labels, and understands all but 1 or 2 relevant main issues and/or problems	Identifies, labels, and understands all relevant main issues and/or problems	
	≤14	15–16	17–18	19–20	Score/Comments
Analysis of issues	Incomplete analysis of the problems/ questions presented in the case	Superficial analysis of some of the problems/questions presented in the case	Thorough analysis of most of the problems/questions presented in the case	Insightful and thorough analysis of all the programs/ questions presented in the case	
	≤14	15–16	17–18	19–20	Score/Comments
Linkage of course readings and other resources to problem/ question	Incomplete or no inquiry into problems/questions with clearly documented linkages to the material read in class, or other assigned resources, previously gained knowledge, and/or outside resources	Limited inquiry into the problems/questions with clearly documented linkages to the material read in class, or other assigned resources, previously gained knowledge, or outside resources	Good inquiry into the problems/questions with clearly documented linkages to the material read in class, and/or other assigned resources, previously gained knowledge, and/or outside resources	Excellent inquiry into the problems/questions with clearly documented linkages to the material read in class, other assigned resources, previously gained knowledge, and outside resources	

	≤14	15–16	17–18	19–20	Score/Comments
Effective response and/or solutions to case study questions	Each response is incorrect, or poorly written, or unreferenced, and irrelevant to question(s) or problem(s) presented	Each response is minimally correct, or well-written, or appropriately referenced, or irrelevant to question(s) or problem(s) presented	Each response is mostly correct, and/or well-written, and/or appropriately referenced, and/or relevant to question(s) and/or problem(s) presented	Each response is correct, well-written, appropriately referenced, and relevant to question(s) or problem(s) presented	

	≤14	15–16	17–18	19–20	Score/Comments
Formatting, spelling, grammar	Multiple errors in APA citations and references. There are multiple mechanical errors such as spelling, formatting, and grammar	May have some errors in APA citations and references. There are some mechanical errors such as spelling, formatting, or grammar	Minimum errors in APA citation and references. There are minimal mechanical errors such as spelling, and/or formatting, and/or grammar	No errors in APA citations or references. There are no mechanical errors such as spelling, formatting, and grammar	

Total points possible: 100	Score and summary comments:

TABLE 11.4   Modifiable Scoring Rubric #2 for a Case Study Assignment

Question #1: (Restate the Question)

	≤ 14	15–16	17–18	19–20	Comments
Effective response and/or solutions to case study questions	Each response is incorrect, or poorly written, or unreferenced, and irrelevant to question(s) or problem(s) presented	Each response is minimally correct, or well-written, or appropriately referenced, or irrelevant to question(s) or problem(s) presented	Each response is mostly correct, and/or well-written, and/or appropriately referenced, and relevant to question(s) and/or problem(s) presented	Each response is correct, well-written, appropriately referenced, and relevant to question(s) or problem(s) presented	
Total points possible: 20/question	**Score and summary comments:**				

TABLE 11.5 Modifiable Scoring Rubric #3 for a Case Study Assignment Using the Nursing Process

	Demonstration of Deeper Understanding and Cognitive Skills				
Criterion	Does Not Meet Expectations ≤ 7	Nearly Meets Expectations 8	Meets Expectations 9	Exceeds Expectations 10	Score and Comments
Interview assessment (10) includes subjective and historical data that support nursing diagnosis	Correctly identifies two clear, specific, and relevant interview (subjective) data points. Data are unorganized, and relevance to nursing diagnosis is unclear.	Correctly identifies three clear, specific, and relevant interview (subjective) data points. Data are marginally organized, and relevance to nursing diagnosis is unclear.	Correctly identifies four clear, specific, and relevant interview (subjective) data points. All data are organized and/or are mostly related to a nursing diagnosis.	Correctly identifies five clear, specific and relevant interview (subjective) data points. All data are organized and are related to a nursing diagnosis.	
Physical assessment (10) includes objective data that support nursing diagnosis	Correctly identifies two clear, specific, and relevant physical (objective) data points. Data are unorganized, and relevance to nursing diagnosis is unclear.	Correctly identifies three clear, specific, and relevant physical (objective) data points. Data are marginally organized, and relevance to nursing diagnosis is unclear.	Correctly identifies four clear, specific, and relevant physical (objective) data points. All data are organized and/or are mostly related to a nursing diagnosis.	Correctly identifies five clear, specific, and relevant physical (objective) data points. All data are organized and are related to a nursing diagnosis.	

(continued)

167

TABLE 11.5 Modifiable Scoring Rubric #3 for a Case Study Assignment Using the Nursing Process (*continued*)

	Demonstration of Deeper Understanding and Cognitive Skills				
Criterion	Does Not Meet Expectations	Nearly Meets Expectations	Meets Expectations	Exceeds Expectations	Score and Comments
	≤7	8	9	10	
Nursing diagnosis (10) Includes relevant NANDA-approved diagnoses written in proper form (includes stem, related to (RT), and as evidenced by (AEB)	Diagnoses are not NANDA approved, appropriate for patient, or not prioritized. Diagnosis may not be clearly supported by assessment data.	Properly identifies two or fewer nursing diagnoses that are clearly supported by the data, and reflect accurate clinical judgment. They may not be appropriate for the patient, well prioritized, NANDA approved, or written in correct format.	Properly identifies three or fewer nursing diagnoses that are clearly supported by the data, and reflect accurate clinical judgment. They are appropriate for the patient, well prioritized, NANDA approved, and written in correct format.	Properly identifies four or more nursing diagnoses that are clearly supported by the data and reflect accurate clinical judgment. They are appropriate for the patient, well prioritized, NANDA approved, and written in correct format.	

	≤ 7	8	9	10
Outcomes / planning (10) including patient and family short- and long-term goals based upon the diagnosis. Goals must be patient focused, realistic, and have clear measurable criteria with a target date/time.	Goal portion is incomplete or completely unrelated to the nursing diagnosis.	Two or fewer short- and long-term goals are identified. Goals may not relate to the nursing diagnosis, may not be written in a patient-focused manner, or are unrealistic. Each goal is missing clear criteria for measurement and a time frame for evaluation.	Three short- and long-term goals are identified that clearly relate to the nursing diagnosis, are written in a patient-focused manner, and are realistic. Each goal contains clear criteria for measurement and a time frame for evaluation.	At least four short- and long-term goals are identified that clearly relate to the nursing diagnosis, are written in a patient-focused manner, and are realistic. Each goal contains clear criteria for measurement and a time frame for evaluation.

(continued)

TABLE 11.5 Modifiable Scoring Rubric #3 for a Case Study Assignment Using the Nursing Process *(continued)*

		Demonstration of Deeper Understanding and Cognitive Skills			
Criterion	Does Not Meet Expectations	Nearly Meets Expectations	Meets Expectations	Exceeds Expectations	Score and Comments
	≤7	8	9	10	
Implementation (10) nursing interventions or actions that directly relate to the etiology of the nursing diagnosis and the patient goal and desired outcome. Each intervention must include referenced rationale (including source and page number if applicable)	Interventions are unclear or do not clearly focus on the etiology of the nursing diagnosis or relate to the patient goals outcomes. Rationales provided do not demonstrate an understanding of the purpose of the interventions or no references are provided.	Identifies fewer than three specific interventions for each outcome criterion related to the etiology of the nursing diagnosis. Not all interventions may be specific. Rationalizations are included but they may be weak, or references are incomplete or from sources that may not be reliable.	Identifies fewer than three specific interventions for each outcome criterion in order to help the patient/family reach the desired goal.	Identifies at least three specific interventions for each outcome criterion in order to help the patient/family reach the desired goal.	

	≤7	8	9	10
Evaluation (10) outlines the methods to be used in evaluating outcome criteria, expectations for goals being met, and what would determine that goal is met, partially met, or unmet. Explain how the plan of care would be revised or continued in each case, including a new realistic evaluation date/time.	Evaluations portion is incomplete or does not relate to diagnosis, goal statement, or interventions.	Evaluation portion does not consistently contain data that are listed as criteria in goal statement. May also not describe goal as met, partially met, or not met. May also not include revision or new evaluation date/time.	Clearly states how each outcome would be evaluated. Able to correctly identify criteria for goal being met, partially met, or unmet. Identifies revisions for care plan but may not include accurate rationale for revision, or references may be from sources that may not be reliable, or a new date is not provided for reevaluation.	Evaluation portion contains data that are listed as criteria in goal statement and lists expectations for meeting the goal. Clear explanation of criteria for goals being met, partially met, or not met. Includes plan for continuation or revision, clearly referenced rationale for revisions from reliable sources, and a new evaluation date/time.

	<7	8	9	10
Identification of the main issues/problems (10)	Unable to identify, label, and understand relevant main issues and/or problems	Identifies, labels, and understands all but three or four relevant main issues and/or problems	Identifies, labels, and understands all but one or two relevant main issues and/or problems	Identifies, labels, and understands all relevant main issues and/or problems

(continued)

TABLE 11.5 Modifiable Scoring Rubric #3 for a Case Study Assignment Using the Nursing Process (*continued*)

		Demonstration of Deeper Understanding and Cognitive Skills			
Criterion	Does Not Meet Expectations	Nearly Meets Expectations	Meets Expectations	Exceeds Expectations	Score and Comments
	<7	8	9	10	
Analysis of issues (10)	Incomplete analysis of the problems/ questions presented in the case	Superficial analysis of some of the problems/questions presented in the case	Thorough analysis of most of the problems/questions presented in the case	Insightful and thorough analysis of all the programs/ questions presented in the case	
	<3.5	3.5	4	5	
Linkage of course readings and other resources to problem/question (5)	Incomplete or no inquiry into problems/questions with clearly documented linkages to the material read in class, other assigned resources, previously gained knowledge, and/or outside resources	Limited inquiry into the problems/ questions with clearly documented linkages to the material read in class, or other assigned resources, previously gained knowledge, or outside resources	Good inquiry into the problems/questions with clearly documented linkages to the material read in class, and/or other assigned resources, previously gained knowledge, and/or outside resources	Excellent inquiry into the problems/ questions with clearly documented linkages to the material read in class, other assigned resources, previously gained knowledge, and outside resources	

	< 3.5	3.5	4	5	Score/Comments
Effective response and/or solutions to case study questions (5)	Each response is incorrect, or poorly written, or unreferenced, and irrelevant to question(s) or problem(s) presented	Each response is minimally correct, well-written or appropriately referenced, or irrelevant to question(s) or problem(s) presented	Each response is mostly correct, or well-written, or appropriately referenced, and relevant to question(s) or problem(s) presented	Each response is correct, well-written, appropriately referenced, and relevant to question(s) or problem(s) presented	

	< 7	8	9	10	Score/Comments
Formatting, spelling, grammar (10)	Multiple errors in APA citations and references. There are multiple mechanical errors such as spelling, formatting, and grammar.	May have some errors in APA citations and references. There are some mechanical errors such as spelling, formatting, and grammar.	Minimum errors in APA citation and references. There are minimal mechanical errors such as spelling, formatting, and grammar.	No errors in APA citations or references. There are no mechanical errors such as spelling, formatting, and grammar.	

Total points possible: 100	Score and summary comments:

Concept Maps

A concept map is a visual tool that represents the individual's interpretation of concepts with integration of past experiences, previous learning, and new knowledge. Gul and Boman (2006) describe concept mapping as a "method of describing ideas about a topic in a picture form" (p. 201). Though concept maps are most typically seen as a teaching/learning strategy, they may also be used for evaluation.

By the end of this chapter, you will learn how to:

- Describe reasons to use concept maps for evaluation
- Discuss the components of a concept map along with the steps for the development of a concept map
- Design a clear assignment description for use of concept maps for evaluation
- Identify prerequisite knowledge and/or resources required by students for a concept map assignment
- Develop or adapt a scoring rubric for concept maps

USING CONCEPT MAPS FOR EVALUATION

Concept maps, as an active teaching/learning strategy, improve critical thinking (Abel & Freeze, 2006; Adema-Hannes & Parzen, 2005; All & Havens, 1999; Clayton, 2006; Daley, Shaw, Balistrieri, Glasenapp, & Piacentine, 1999; Vacek, 2009; Wheeler & Collins, 2003; Wilgis & McConnell, 2008) and knowledge retention (Li-Ling, 2004; Nesbit & Adesope, 2006). They also facilitate deep learning (Daley et al., 1999) and improve clinical judgment and decision making (Beitz, 1998; Gerdeman, Luz, & Jacko, 2012). Concept maps contribute to the processes of scaffolding new knowledge to prior knowledge, organization of information logically, prioritization, and retention of knowledge (Adema-Hannes & Parzen, 2005; Li-Ling, 2004). Concept maps also encourage creativity and divergent thinking.

Although there have been few studies to evaluate the use of concept maps for summative evaluation, concept maps prove to be valuable in assessing students' knowledge. Concept maps allow evaluation of Bloom's higher cognitive levels such as analyzing, evaluating, and creating (Luckowski, 2003). Concept maps are useful to demonstrate analysis, synthesis, and prioritization. They require the student to have a global grasp of a situation with synthesis of new and old knowledge rather than just remembering (King & Shell, 2002; Mueller, Johnson, & Bligh, 2002). Also, faculty are able to easily recognize a student's misconception through the use of a concept map.

Educators frequently use concept mapping in place of traditional care plans for preparation and evaluation in clinical courses. Taylor and Littleton-Kearney (2011) used concept maps along with case-study clinical rounds with advanced practice nursing students. While several students complained about the time required to develop the concept maps, other student comments supported the positive impact on critical thinking.

There are some disadvantages to the use of concept mapping for evaluation. They are time-consuming and many students do not know anything about the process (Beitz, 1998). Concept maps are most appropriate for visual learners, while linear thinkers may have difficulty with what they may perceive as the chaos (Hill, 2006; Mueller et al., 2001). Use of concept maps may be a difficult leap for students accustomed to traditional learning methods (Quinn, Mintzes, & Laws, 2004). However, Kostovich, Poradzisz, Wood, and O'Brien (2007) found no relationship between learning style preference, using Kolb's four learning styles, and a student's grade on a concept map assignment. While it is recognized and accepted that learners do have a preference for learning styles, it is also recognized that use of a variety of teaching/learning strategies is beneficial to the student (Brookfield, 1987; Loo, 2004).

The components of a concept map are concepts, relationships, and crosslinks. Holliday (2013) and Toofany (2008), and others have provided simple step-by-step processes for creating a concept map. This process of developing a concept map begins with contemplation, data collection, and listing of concepts. Concept mapping starts with a central concept in the form of a word or phrase. Other concepts, descriptive words, aspects, and questions associated with the central concept are listed and then grouped and arranged hierarchically around the central concept. The linking of concepts with relationships or potential relationships occurs next. The lines that link the concepts include prepositions or linking words, such as "causes," "leads to," "is associated with," or "occurs with," to indicate the nature of the relationship between concepts. Finally, a look at the entire concept map identifies any missing concepts or relationships. A concept map of a concept map is included as Figure 12.1.

WRITING THE ASSIGNMENT DESCRIPTION

The most important aspect of the assignment description is the purpose of the concept map and the relationship of the purpose to the course objectives. So, as always, begin with information about the effects of concept maps on deep learning and critical thinking. This is likely the first time the student will be asked to do a concept map. You will likely need to provide an explanation of what a concept map is and how it can (1) help the student learn and (2) allow you to evaluate what the student understands about the assignment topic.

Most likely you will ask students to do a concept map related to a key content area of the course. Concept maps are very helpful in pathophysiology (e.g., pathophysiologic conditions), didactic

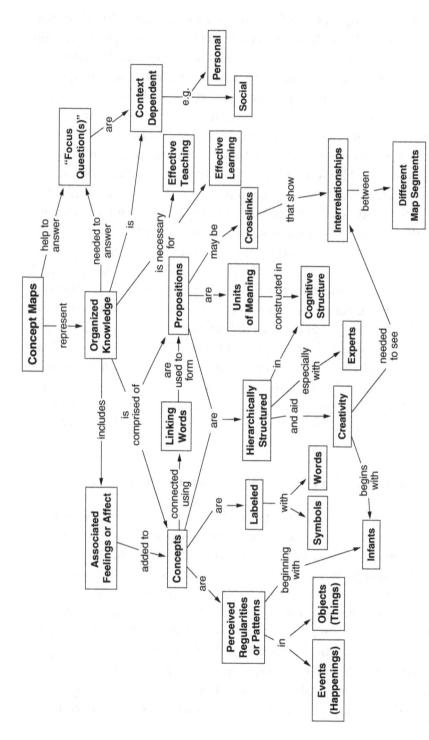

FIGURE 12.1 Concept map of a concept map.

Source: Novak and Canas (2008).

nursing courses (e.g., medical or nursing diagnoses), or clinical nursing courses (e.g., the student's assigned patient), but they can also be used in management or leadership courses (e.g., issues). If students are to choose a topic, list possible choices. If students will determine their own topic, include a deadline for submission of the topic for your approval.

Be specific about your expectations for the concept map such as how many levels you expect or what key areas you expect to be included. For example, in pathophysiology, you may expect etiology, clinical presentation, diagnostic studies, and collaborative management, including medical and nursing treatments. Identify the expected size of the concept map and the font size in the map. Be clear about how citations are to be done. Consider asking that the citations be numbered sequentially and the corresponding number superscripted in the box.

The map can be pasted into a Word document behind the title page and before the reference page. Specify how and when the map is due. Most likely you will want an electronic version delivered either to the assignment manager in your learning management system or by e-mail.

Clinical Pearl

There are many different software options available for developing concept maps. While it is not necessary that everyone use the same software to develop the map, the assignment should be submitted as either a Word document or a PDF with the map embedded. It is best to specify which format (i.e., Word or PDF) you want.

IDENTIFYING PRIOR KNOWLEDGE AND/OR RESOURCES TO BE AVAILABLE FOR STUDENTS

Since this is likely to be the first time the student will be asked to develop a concept map, you will need to provide a thorough explanation regarding what a concept map is and how to develop one.

You might even provide an example such as the "concept map of a concept map" included as Figure 12.1.

You will need to provide guidance regarding methods of map development. The concepts initially may either be listed on a piece of paper or on sticky notes. This can be developed on a piece of paper or on a wall with the sticky notes. While students may develop concept maps with pen and paper or sticky notes, those methods should not be accepted as the final product because legibility is usually inadequate. Word or PowerPoint can be used but there are also special software programs specific to concept maps. The following is a list of links to some of these programs; these are all either free or have a free trial version available.

- cmap.ihmc.us/download
- www.inspiration.com/freetrial
- www.smartdraw.com
- www.xmind.net
- www.edrawsoft.com/ConceptMap.php

Include directives if you want specific areas to be a specific color. Identify if you want some concepts to be a specific shape. For instance, in a pathophysiology course where you have assigned a pathologic condition, you may want pathophysiology to be one shape or color and the clinical presentation to be another shape or color, and so forth. Also, specify how many levels or areas you expect.

Students need resources on American Psychological Association (APA) style for their references. If you do not require that they buy the APA manual, you may consider providing the URL for Owl Purdue Online Writing Lab (owl.english.purdue.edu/owl/resource/560/01) in the assignment description.

MODIFYING FOR ONLINE DELIVERY

There is no modification necessary for this assignment but it is likely that you will want students to be able to share the concept maps that they developed. You will want to specify the file type, which is most likely to be PDF or Word, and how you want the file named, such as LASTNAMECONCEPTMAP.

EVALUATING THE CONCEPT MAP

Concept maps can be difficult to score. They are best viewed on a large monitor using the zoom function to focus into areas sequentially. Modify the following scoring rubric (Table 12.1) as necessary. Return the concept map with comments along with the rubric pasted at the bottom of the paper.

CONCLUSION

Concept maps can be a fun and interesting way to demonstrate knowledge of a topic. Concept maps can be developed using pencil and paper, Word, PowerPoint, or other specific concept map software programs, so students do need guidance if they have never developed a concept map. While they may be technically challenging, many students will excel at development of a concept map and find the learning enjoyable.

TABLE 12.1 Modifiable Scoring Rubric for Concept Map Assignment

Criterion (Points Possible)	Does Not Meet Expectations ≤14	Nearly Meets Expectations 15–16	Meets Expectations 17–18	Exceeds Expectations 19–20	Score and Comments
Accuracy (20)	The map includes many minor or major errors or misconceptions. Inaccurate on many key concepts.	The map contains several minor errors or at least one major error or misconception but is accurate on most key concepts.	The map contains only a few minor errors but is accurate on all key concepts.	The map contains no errors or misconceptions.	
Comprehensiveness (20)	The map demonstrates only superficial knowledge of the topic. The map contains hardly any key concepts, and those that are presented are not developed.	The map demonstrates moderate knowledge of the topic. The map contains only a few key concepts and those presented are weakly developed.	The map demonstrates good knowledge of the topic. The map contains most key concepts but does not demonstrate complex thinking.	The map demonstrates in-depth knowledge of the topic. The map contains all key concepts. Complex thinking about the central concept is evident.	

	≤ 14	15–16	17–18	19–20
Organization and structure (20)	The map is generally linear or disorganized. The map fails to demonstrate connections among concepts. It is difficult to identify the central concept. The map is difficult to read.	The map is nonlinear but the concepts and links are difficult to follow. The map demonstrates only a few connections among concepts. Many linking words are omitted or inappropriate. Most of the map is difficult to read.	The map is nonlinear. The concepts and links are easy to follow and understand. The map demonstrates most connections among concepts. A few linking words are omitted or inappropriate. Most of the map is clearly legible.	The map is nonlinear and treelike. Concepts and links are easy to follow and understand. The map demonstrates all appropriate connections among concepts and linking words accurately describe relationships. The map is clearly legible.

	≤ 14	15–16	17–18	19–20
Sources (20)	The concept map is based solely on personal opinion, lay literature, or commercial websites. There are multiple errors in APA citations and references.	The concept map is based on references limited to textbooks or commercial (e.g., .com) websites. There are several errors in APA citations and references.	The concept map is based on multiple references, including material from professional journals and noncommercial (e.g., .gov, .edu, .org) websites. At least two current research articles are included in references. There are only one or two minor errors in APA citations or references.	The concept map is based on multiple (more than 10) references, including material from professional journals and noncommercial (e.g., .gov, .edu, .org) websites. Multiple current research articles are included in references. There are no errors in APA citations or references.

(continued)

TABLE 12.1 Modifiable Scoring Rubric for Concept Map Assignment (*continued*)

Criterion (Points Possible)	Does Not Meet Expectations	Nearly Meets Expectations	Meets Expectations	Exceeds Expectations	Score and Comments
	≤ 14	15–16	17–18	19–20	
Creativity (20)	The concept map shows limited or no creativity.	The concept map illustrates minimal creativity in layout, use of shapes, use of color, or interconnectedness. Color is used primarily for aesthetics rather than clarity.	The concept map illustrates creativity in layout, use of shapes, use of color, and interconnectedness. Color is used to improve clarity.	The concept map illustrates creativity in layout, use of shapes, use of color, and interconnectedness. Color is used to improve clarity. Appropriate visual and/or audio embeds enhance concept map.	
Total points possible: 100	**Score and summary comments:**				

Posters

As educators, we are very familiar with posters and poster presentations as a source of presenting and disseminating valuable information and scholarship at professional nursing conferences. Indeed, the utilization of posters and poster presentations at nursing conferences dates as far back as the early 1970s (Wharrad, Allcock, & Meal, 1995). Since then, posters gained the respect of our profession, and are an expected and well-received alternative to podium presentations in conferences around the world.

This chapter discusses how posters and poster presentation assignments can be utilized in student evaluation. Advantages and disadvantages to using posters for student evaluation are considered, and guidelines for assignment description creation are presented.

By the end of this chapter, you will learn how to:

- Describe reasons to use posters and poster presentations for evaluation
- Design a clear assignment description for posters for evaluation

- Identify prerequisite knowledge and/or resources required by students for a poster assignment
- Adapt a poster assignment of online courses
- Develop or adapt a scoring rubric for a poster assignment
- Consider the involvement of students in the peer evaluation of presentations

USING POSTERS AND POSTER PRESENTATIONS FOR EVALUATION

As a viable alternative to test taking and paper writing, the utilization of posters as a teaching and learning strategy and evaluation method is gaining popularity. Evidence of their utilization can be found across all levels and types of nursing programs. For example, students in undergraduate nursing courses may be assigned to create posters to gain a deeper understanding of concepts reviewed in class or read in the required text. When they present this information in a poster format to their peers, those fellow students learn more deeply, and may more likely remember vital information from this creative and visual display (Wharrad et al., 1995). Wharrad et al. (1995) assert, "The sharing of knowledge at a more personal level can be beneficial to both teachers and students. The need for . . . brevity and article imagery when preparing a good poster means the viewer is left with a mental image of the information which is more likely to be retained and recalled later" (p. 370).

Graduate nursing programs also incorporate poster development assignments throughout their curricula (Christenbery & Latham, 2013). Typically, these posters are focused on the presentation of scholarship (Christenbery & Latham, 2013). For example, PhD students may present the results of their research (finished or in progress) and DNP students may present their projects in a poster format to elicit feedback from their student colleagues and educators (Christenbery & Latham, 2013).

Regardless of the student's academic level (undergraduate or graduate), or type of poster created, the benefits of utilizing posters for student evaluation in academia are many. Using posters for evaluation gives students an opportunity to:

- Develop communication skills and boost confidence (Christenbery & Latham, 2013)

- Interact with other student colleagues and professors with provision of an opportunity to discuss their topic, or answer questions about their research, and to expand on poster content (Christenbery & Latham, 2013)

- Develop critical thinking (O'Neill & Jennings, 2012) and networking skills (Christenbery & Latham, 2013)

- Be involved in the assessment process (O'Neill & Jennings, 2012)

- Investigate a topic thoroughly (O'Neill & Jennings, 2012)

- Learn from their peers (O'Neill & Jennings, 2012)

- Gain valuable feedback from peers and educators

- Explore and confront misconceptions (O'Neill & Jennings, 2012)

- Learn visually (Summers, 2005)

- Practice professional poster development and presentations for ongoing use in their professional field (Wharrad et al., 1995)

Clinical Pearl

There are many advantages to utilizing posters for student evaluation in nursing programs, including the opportunity for students to learn from their peers, develop critical thinking, and obtain valuable feedback from their peers and educators.

Some disadvantages to using posters for student evaluation include:

- Poster development is new to most students, requiring detailed instruction
- Posters take considerable time to develop, and space for presentation of printed posters may be an issue (Summers, 2005)
- Assessment rubrics are sometimes unclear about expectations, creating a concern for interrater reliability (Summers, 2005)
- Posters can be expensive to produce (Siegrist, Garett-Wright, & Abel, 2011) if you plan to have them actually printed

WRITING THE ASSIGNMENT DESCRIPTION

When creating a poster assignment description, develop specific guidelines that provide students the parameters of the assignment, and the opportunity for students to work on it independently (Moule, Judd, & Girot, 1998). These guidelines should describe and clarify the following assignment elements:

- **Linkage to one or more course objectives**.
- **Placement in curriculum.** Determine where the poster assignment will be placed within the student's curriculum. Will this be an assignment in one particular course, or will the poster and its contents be developed over multiple courses within the student's program of study? Might this assignment be a program requirement and not attached to any particular course?
- **Selection of topics.** If students are not presenting their scholarship, determine if they will be assigned or be able to select from a group of preapproved topics. Consider requiring an abstract, which contains the essential elements of a poster, early on in the development process.
- **Working alone or in groups.** Determine if students will work alone or in small groups. If working in groups, determine if

students will have an opportunity to evaluate each other's performance in the development of the poster. A peer evaluation form is available.

- **Evaluation.** Determine if the assignment evaluation feedback will be formative, providing constructive feedback only, or summative (for a grade). Determine to what extent student peers will be part of the evaluation process.

- **Reason for the poster assignment.** Clarify the reason for the poster assignment (e.g., review of information, dissemination of research, etc.), and determine if the assignment also requires the student to participate in a poster presentation.

- **Poster template.** Provide students with a poster template. At the very least, this template should include specifics about the names of major section headings, and a brief description of each section. Remind students that posters are designed to present, in a creatively visual way, only *the most important information* they want the reader to understand. Posters should be eye-catching, and readable in less than 5 minutes (Bischof, 2013). Encourage students to save their final poster in an unalterable file format such as .PDF.

- **Poster medium.** Determine the medium in which the poster will be presented. Will the students be required to print the poster onto poster board or develop an e-poster to be disseminated electronically? Will the poster be displayed at a particular venue for others to review (i.e., a classroom, hall, or conference room)?

- **Poster layout parameters.** Describe the parameters of the poster layout, including size, number of sections, and the use of color, font, and text.

- **Poster software.** Clarify which software can be utilized in developing the poster assignment (e.g., Microsoft PowerPoint or other Internet resource).

- **Evidence-based practice (EBP) poster.** If you are creating an EBP poster assignment for MSN or DNP students, consider requiring the following poster layout headings (Table 13.1):

TABLE 13.1   Comparison of Headers for Posters

Headings of an EBP Poster	Headings of a Research Poster
Banner and title	Banner and title
Introduction	Introduction
Clinical problem and key objectives (i.e., PICOT question)	Aims, objectives, and/or research question(s)/hypotheses
A brief description of the patients, setting, and scholarly project	Methods
Outcomes and clinical relevance	Findings
Conclusion and recommendations for practice	Conclusion
References	References

(1) banner and title; (2) introduction; (3) the project's clinical problem and key objectives (i.e., PICOT question); (4) a brief description of the patients, setting, and scholarly project; (5) outcomes and clinical relevance; (6) the conclusion and recommendations for practice; and (7) references (Christenbery & Latham, 2013).

- **Research poster.** If you are creating a research poster assignment for students (e.g., PhD), consider requiring the common research-related poster layout headings (Table 13.1): (1) banner and title; (2) introduction; (3) aims, objective, background and/or research question(s)/hypotheses; (4) methods; (5) findings; (6) conclusion; and (7) references.

PRIOR KNOWLEDGE AND RESOURCES TO BE AVAILABLE TO STUDENTS

To be successful developing and presenting posters, students must understand the basic fundamentals of poster development. It is important for educators to provide detailed instructions (in addition to assignment description and guidelines) regarding how to create a professional poster. Provide students with examples and a poster template, if possible. Bischoff (2013) provides a variety of Internet resources from which students can select their own poster templates to develop professional-quality posters (Box 13.1). An easy alternative to these web sources is to provide students with a pre-approved Microsoft PowerPoint template.

BOX 13.1

Poster Printing Sites

Quark Software, Inc. www.quark.com

PhD Posters phdposters.com

Graphicsland, Inc. www.makesigns.com

SciGen Technologies www.postergenius.com/cms/index.php

P & D Display Graphics, LLC posters4research.com

MegaPrint, Inc. www.postersession.com

PosterPresentations.com www.posterpresentations.com

SciFor, Inc. www.scifor.com

Adapted from Bischof (2013).

Clinical Pearl

To be successful developing and presenting posters, students must understand the basic fundamentals of poster development. Students will benefit from poster creation and printing websites. Consider giving students a preapproved PowerPoint template.

MODIFYING THE ASSIGNMENT FOR ONLINE USE

For online courses and programs, assigning students to develop posters, and even present, is similar to an on-campus assignment. When assigning a poster and/or poster presentation in an online course, consider altering the following assignment guidelines.

Poster medium. The poster medium is limited to electronic submission in online courses/programs. Remind students to submit their final e-poster in an unalterable final format, such as .PDF. Students can submit their e-posters via e-mail or through the learning management system. If submitting through a learning management system, peer and educator review, and time for answering questions, are encouraged. For example, the student can submit his or her e-poster into a forum on Blackboard where colleagues and educators can learn from, dialogue, and ask questions about its content. Some schools may also have the ability for students to present their e-posters through teleconferencing software such as Adobe Connect or Blackboard Collaborate.

EVALUATING THE POSTER ASSIGNMENT

Evaluating a poster can be challenging, especially when submitted electronically. It is helpful to look at the poster in its entirety and then section by section using the zoom function. The following scoring rubric (Table 13.2) can be modified as needed. Return the rubric to the student with comments.

TABLE 13.2 Modifiable Scoring Rubric for Poster Assignment

Criterion (Points Possible)	Does Not Meet Expectations	Nearly Meets Expectations	Meets Expectations	Exceeds Expectations	Score and Comments
	≤7	8	9	10	
Layout/ organization (10)	Information is displayed in a disorganized manner. Appropriate headings are not used. Sections of the poster are not separated by space with no text or graphics. There is no sequence to the display of information. Title and author and affiliations are omitted.	Information is displayed in a somewhat disorganized manner. Some appropriate headings used. Sections of the poster are poorly separated by space with no text or graphics. There is no sequence to the display of information. Title or author or author affiliations are omitted.	Information is displayed in a somewhat organized manner. Appropriate headings are used. Sections of the poster are separated by space with no text or graphics. There is a sequence to the display of information but it is not immediately obvious. Title and author and affiliations are evident.	Information is displayed in an organized manner. Appropriate headings are used. Sections of the poster are separated by space with no text or graphics. There is an obvious sequence to the display of information. Title, author, and affiliations are clearly evident.	

(continued)

TABLE 13.2 Modifiable Scoring Rubric for Poster Assignment (continued)

Criterion (Points Possible)	Does Not Meet Expectations	Nearly Meets Expectations	Meets Expectations	Exceeds Expectations	Score and Comments
	≤ 28	29–32	33–36	37–40	
Content discussion of assigned topic With required content (40) (*List required content here*)	Poster omitted required content. Lack of even basic knowledge of topic evident through poster. Poster is of no educational benefit.	Poster did include required content but superficial and/or several inaccuracies noted. Superficial knowledge of the topic evident through poster. Poster is of little educational benefit.	Poster of assigned topic with required content at appropriate depth and detail. Some minor inaccuracies noted. Knowledge of the topic is evident through poster. Poster is educational for others.	Exemplary poster of assigned topic with required content at appropriate depth, detail, and accuracy within the space restrictions of a poster. Extensive knowledge of the topic is clearly evident through poster. Poster is educational for others.	
	≤ 14	15–16	17–18	19–20	
Use of scientific evidence (20)	No discussion of the scientific evidence. References listed fewer than five references. Multiple errors in American Psychological Association (APA) citations and references.	Limited discussion of scientific evidence related to topic. References list includes at least five to seven references with fewer than three of these research studies. More than two errors in APA citations and references.	Good discussion of scientific evidence related to topic. Reference list includes at least eight references with at least three of these high-quality research studies. No more than two errors in APA citations or references.	Exemplary discussion of the scientific evidence related to topic. Reference list includes at least 10 references with at least five high-quality research studies cited. No errors in APA citations or references.	

	≤ 14	15–16	17–18	19–20
Visual presentation (20)	Many errors in spelling, word usage, or punctuation. Font selection and/or size inappropriate. Use of distracting colors or visuals. Distracting graphics or inadequate graphics. No creativity demonstrated. Text is not legible at five feet if physical poster or on 19-inch monitor at 18 inches if computer format.	More than two errors in spelling, word usage, or punctuation. Font selection and/or size inappropriate. Distracting colors or poor contrast. Distracting graphics or inadequate graphics. Little creativity demonstrated. Only some text is legible at five feet if physical poster or on 19-inch monitor at 18 inches if computer format.	No more than two errors in spelling, word usage, or punctuation. Font size and/or selection appropriate. Good use of color and contrast. Use of graphics slightly less than or more than appropriate. Some creativity. Most of text is legible at five feet if physical poster or on 19-inch monitor at 18 inches if computer format.	No errors in spelling, word usage, or punctuation. Font size and/or selection appropriate. Good use of color and contrast. Appropriate use of only relevant graphics. Exemplary creativity demonstrated. Text is legible at five feet if physical poster or on 19-inch monitor at 18 inches if computer format.

(continued)

TABLE 13.2 Modifiable Scoring Rubric for Poster Assignment (*continued*)

Criterion (Points Possible)	Does Not Meet Expectations	Nearly Meets Expectations	Meets Expectations	Exceeds Expectations	Score and Comments
	≤7	8	9	10	
Poster presentation (10) (if verbal presentation included; if not, add these points to content)	Casual attire. Student failed to introduce self and reason for interest in topic. Frequent pauses, lots of uhs, hmmms, or you knows, or monotone. Speech is too soft, too loud, too fast, or too slow. Limited vocabulary and frequent mispronunciations. Use of slang or profanity. Almost exclusively reading from poster or notes. Does not look at audience, move, or smile. Distracting mannerisms. More than 20% over time limit.	Casual attire. Student introduced self but omitted reason for interest in topic. Hesitancy, some uhs, hmmms, or you knows. Limited variation in intonation. Speech is too soft, too loud, too fast, or too slow. Limited vocabulary and more than two mispronunciations. Use of slang or profanity. Frequently reads from poster or notes. Rarely looks at audience. Stiff body movements. Does not smile. More than 10% over time limit.	Professional attire. Student introduced self and reason for interest in topic. No hesitancy or uhs, hmmms, or you knows. Does vary intonation and speech is of appropriate loudness and speed. Good vocabulary and no more than 1–2 mispronunciations. No use of slang or profanity. Uses notes minimally and does not read from poster. Occasionally looks at audience members. Uses some hand gestures. Smiles when appropriate. No more than 10% over time limit.	Professional attire. Student introduced self and reason for interest in topic. Enthusiastic and engaging. Speech is fluid with clear enunciation. Uses voice to communicate interest by varying intonation and appropriate loudness and speed. Excellent vocabulary with no mispronunciations. No use of slang or profanity. No reading from poster. Establishes eye contact with audience; scans room. Natural hand gestures. Smiles when appropriate. Adheres to time limit.	

Total points possible: 100	**Score and summary comments:**

CONCLUSION

The profession of nursing is very accustomed to the use of posters and poster presentations at professional conferences. A lessor-known fact, posters and poster presentations are excellent student evaluation tools, and are viable alternatives to test taking, paper writing, and other assignments. Using posters for evaluation gives students an opportunity to develop communication skills and boost confidence, interact with colleagues, develop critical thinking, and gain valuable feedback from peers and educators. Disadvantages of using posters for student evaluation are minimal and include considerable time to develop, cost, and the difficulty creating a clear list of assignment expectations. To aid educators, this chapter presented guidelines for writing the poster and poster presentation assignment description. Lastly, educators can modify and use the scoring rubric for poster evaluation outlined in Table 13.2.

Student Portfolios

A portfolio is defined as "collections of evidence used by an individual to document specific achievements, competencies, and learning outcomes" (Hawks, 2012, p. 90). A student portfolio is a unique collection of student-maintained materials that demonstrates student growth, learning, and development over a designated period of time. This portfolio provides a mechanism for the student to track and reflect on academic experiences, assignments, and competencies while safely exploring professional roles, responsibilities, and interests. A student portfolio provides students an opportunity to highlight their academic accomplishments, and may be maintained to plan and facilitate a successful transition into a professional role (Friedrich et al., 2010; FriWassef, Riza, Maciag, Worden, & Delaney, 2012; Hawks, 2012; Head & Johnson, 2012; McColgan & Blackwood, 2009; Rossettiet al., 2012). This chapter focuses on the development and use of a portfolio as an assignment and a method of evaluation of the student's level of achievement of the specific course learning objectives and/or program outcomes.

By the end of this chapter, you will learn how to:

- Describe reasons to use a portfolio for evaluation

- Design a clear assignment description for portfolios for evaluation

- Identify prerequisite knowledge and/or resources required by students for developing a portfolio

- Develop or adapt a scoring rubric for evaluation of a portfolio

USING PORTFOLIOS FOR EVALUATION

Portfolios are being used increasingly in undergraduate and graduate nursing programs (Friedrich et al., 2010; FriWassef et al., 2012; Hawks, 2012; Head & Johnson, 2012; McColgan & Blackwood, 2009; McMullen et al., 2003; Rossetti et al., 2012). Portfolios allow the student and the educator to assess and evaluate achievement of learning objectives, reflect on learning progress, as well as identify continued learning needs (Rosetti et al., 2012). The student portfolio reflects the personal and professional products of the learning process. Select graded assignments are kept in the portfolio and the students are encouraged to reflect on the learning that has occurred as well as on the potential implications for that learning. A student's portfolio is intended to show the reviewer the level of growth, competencies, and professional achievement attained during the specified time (FriWassef et al., 2012; Hawks, 2012). A portfolio can be developed for use within a specific course or be maintained across a curriculum of study. When used across the curriculum, the portfolio provides a tangible outcome that can be refined and transitioned into a professional portfolio as students move into professional settings.

The use of portfolios as an assignment in nursing education is based in adult learning theory (Hawks, 2010; McMullan et al., 2003; Rossetti et al., 2012). Assumptions for the development and use of a portfolio include that the student is self-directed and ready to learn, and will do so through learning experiences and reflection on these experiences (Bastable, 2014; Byrne, Schroeter, Carter, & Mower, 2009;

Friedrich et al., 2010; McMullan et al., 2003). The process of completing a portfolio requires the student to integrate knowledge in a manner that results in the student demonstrating achievement of the learning outcome(s). This may be done through documentation of skills and competencies, reflection on learning that has occurred, and the completion and collection of other assignments and materials that demonstrate learning. In addition, gaps in learning are easier to identify (FriWassef et al., 2012; Hawks, 2010). The process of creating and maintaining a portfolio promotes students':

- Integration of theory and practice (McMullan et al., 2003)
- Awareness of their competencies, skills, strengths, and limitations (McMullan et al., 2003)
- Personal development (Head & Johnson, 2012; McMullan et al., 2003)
- Responsibility for their own learning (McMullan et al., 2003)
- Professional identity and goal setting (Hawk, 2010; McColgan & Blackwood, 2009)
- Organization and structure (Head & Johnson, 2012)
- Communication (McMullan et al., 2003)

Concerns identified about the use of portfolios include that they can be:

- Difficult and time-consuming to develop (Head & Johnson, 2012)
- Repetitive (Head & Johnson, 2012)
- Cumbersome when maintained in hard copy (FriWassef et al., 2012)

If the portfolio is an assignment in a capstone course or intended as an end-of-program assignment to document achievement of program outcomes, materials may be arranged in folders corresponding to the end-of-program outcomes or the American Association of Colleges of Nursing (AACN) Essentials for the program. These folders can be tabs in an actual notebook or electronic file folders in an e-portfolio. These folders should include a student narrative of how they achieved the outcome or essential statement with supporting evidence, such as papers or project descriptions.

Students' portfolios lay the foundation for a professional portfolio. Encourage students to continue to add to their portfolios as they move into their professional roles. This will provide a centralized and organized vehicle for maintaining information that is often required for licensure, credentialing, and continuing academic pursuits (Oermann, 2002).

WRITING THE ASSIGNMENT DESCRIPTION

Clearly identify the need for and purpose of the portfolio. Typically this is included in the course syllabus. Specifically, identify how the required elements in the portfolio relate to achievement of the course learning objectives and more broadly the programmatic outcomes. Consider which course products provide the best opportunity to demonstrate achievement of the course learning objectives, as this ultimately is the rationale for selecting that element to be part of the student's portfolio. Within the portfolio there should be opportunity for student reflection on the assignment, as well as evaluation of the assignment. While reflection is an essential component of a student portfolio, this may be an area that the student may not want to share in a professional setting.

In schools where the portfolio is maintained throughout the curriculum, across classes and instructors, it is imperative there is a universal understanding among educators of how the portfolio is structured and maintained. This helps avoid confusion and frustration for students and educators due to varying expectations. Depending on where the course you are teaching is situated in the curriculum, this assignment may include initiating the e-portfolio, or simply working within and adding to an active e-portfolio document.

Key Components of the Portfolio

Portfolios by nature are individual and thus may all look different in terms of colors and font used, supporting visuals and various individual preferences in terms of layout of pages. Colors and visuals are used to individualize and enhance the portfolio. Advise students to avoid color combinations or pictures that overwhelm or detract from the content or make the information in the portfolio difficult to read. The focus of the portfolio is to present the information in an organized and polished manner.

Regardless of the format, the expected content, structure, and use of the portfolio needs to be uniform for students and clearly articulated. Expectations for the key components of the portfolio as specified in Box 14.1 need to be clear and contain specific direction as to what is required and within what time frame. These expectations serve as the guideline for the scoring rubric.

BOX 14.1

Components of a Portfolio

Title page
Table of contents

1. Student information

   - Student name

   - Picture

   - Contact information: e-mail, phone, address

   - Name of school

   - Expected graduation date

2. Resume/CV

3. Professional documents

   - Cover letter

   - Letters of recommendation

4. Career path

5. Copy of each course syllabus, followed by the required student work product(s) with evaluation and student reflection regarding the assignments

6. Self-assessments: Strengths, weaknesses, competencies

Portfolio Format

A portfolio can be developed and maintained in a hard copy or electronic format. A hard copy portfolio can be created with a three-ring binder, with tabbed section dividers to facilitate organization and ease of maneuvering through the binder. A table of contents should be provided so it is clear where the required information is located for ease of use and evaluation. Encourage the student to secure all items in the binder. An electronic copy of the hard copy documents allows for easy revisions as necessary, and provides a backup in case the hard copy gets damaged or lost. All documents in the portfolio should be clear, easy to read, and free of dirt and stains. Page protectors are excellent to preserve the integrity of the portfolio documents in the binder. While it may be nice to have a hard copy, a portfolio in this format can quickly result in a lot of paper that can be overwhelming, cumbersome to transport, and more difficult to update.

An e-portfolio is a portfolio that is developed and maintained in an electronic format. Maintaining an e-portfolio can reduce paper load; increase ease of storage through use of a flash drive, shared drive, or cloud; and increase portability and accessibility of portfolio documents (FriWassef et al., 2012). Accessibility needs to be ensured for the student and the educator in the locations where it will be needed. Creating and using an e-portfolio may be a new process for the student and educator, which can be overwhelming. It may be helpful, as the educator, to create an e-portfolio to facilitate a working knowledge of this type of assignment.

How to Create an E-Portfolio

There are many electronic platforms that support development of an e-portfolio. These include sites such as: www.weebly.com, www.wix.com, www.yola.com, and www.prezi.com. Also, many academic platforms support development of e-portfolios. Check with your academic institution's information technology (IT) department to explore how e-portfolios may be supported. Logistically, as the educator, it simplifies the evaluation process if the students use the same program for their e-portfolios. Caution students to avoid using platforms that charge a fee for their service, as this may require the viewer to also pay the fee in order to view the e-portfolio.

Required Elements of the Portfolio

Be clear about required elements of the portfolio; these will be used in the development of the grading rubric. Link the portfolio assignment to specific course student-learning objectives or program-learning outcomes. Specify competencies or learning objectives that will be assessed through the use of the portfolio. Talk about the process of self-directed learning, reflection, and the process of growth. The process of identifying personal limitations and areas that need improvement can be threatening for students who have not done this in the past. The idea behind the academic portfolio is that it provides a structure for the student to use to become a self-directed lifetime learner. It also provides a structure for the student to keep track of and organize his or her accomplishments, and clarify professional goals as the student moves into a professional position.

Describe how the portfolio is expected to look and how it will be used in addition to any specific expectations with respect to how the portfolio will be reviewed. Within the first 2 weeks of the semester, make sure that the structure for the portfolio is established. If a hard copy is being used, it may be helpful to have the student submit the binder, with dividers that specify the required elements. If the portfolio is being managed electronically, have the student establish the portfolio on the designated site, complete at least one page, and provide the access information to the educator to ensure the portfolio is easily accessible by someone other than the student. This prevents last-minute student procrastination and provides ample opportunity to correct any misunderstandings or difficulties in setup and access of the student's portfolio.

IDENTIFYING PRIOR KNOWLEDGE AND/OR RESOURCES TO BE AVAILABLE FOR STUDENTS

For a hard copy portfolio, the student will need a binder, tabbed divider sheets, and possibly sheet protectors. Basic computer skills will be necessary to develop the hard copies of the information. For an e-portfolio, the student will need access to a network platform that supports e-portfolios. As identified above, several are available free of charge. Caution students who are considering paying for access to a service. This may create a problem, as those who need to access the portfolio may also have to join that service for a fee. Establish from the start that, as the educator, access to the e-portfolio needs to be free of charge.

MODIFYING FOR ONLINE DELIVERY

An e-portfolio is well suited for online delivery and educator review. The e-portfolio stored on a hard drive or flash drive can be e-mailed or sent to a designated space in the electronic course management system. As these can be large files, it may be necessary to condense the file into a zip file for easier online delivery. For a web-based e-portfolio, the student should provide the link or web address for easy access. Remind students to check that privacy or security settings, either applied or part of the website, do not prevent access or review by the educator.

Evaluating a Portfolio

A rubric that highlights and describes the key components and presentation expectations for the portfolio should be developed. This is particularly valuable when the portfolio is being maintained by students throughout their program and is an assignment and evaluation method across courses. An example of a rubric for a student portfolio is provided in Table 14.1. Modify the rubric as needed and use it to score the student portfolio. Return the completed rubric electronically either by e-mail as an attachment or through the assignment

TABLE 14.1 Modifiable Scoring Rubric for a Portfolio Assignment

Category (Points Possible)	Does Not Meet Expectations	Nearly Meets Expectations	Meets Expectations	Exceeds Expectations	Comments
	≤ 10	11–12	13–14	15	
Portfolio organization and structure (15)	**Hard copy:** The documents are not bound or the binder is too large or small for the contents or there are documents in the binder that are not secured. One or more of the required sections are missing or disorganized. The table of contents is missing.	**Hard copy:** The documents are all secured in an appropriately sized binder that allows the reader to easily review the contents. All of the required sections are present but there is some disorganization with some documents being misfiled. The table of contents is incomplete or does not adequately direct the reviewer to the appropriate section.	**Hard copy:** The documents are all secured in an appropriately sized binder that allows the reader to easily review the contents. All of the required sections are present with at least one piece of supporting documentation in each. The table of contents is organized and directs the reviewer to the appropriate section.	**Hard copy:** The documents are all secured in an appropriately sized binder that allows the reader to easily review the contents. All of the required sections are separated by tabbed dividers that are clearly labeled, and contain multiple sources of supporting documentation. The table of contents is organized and directs the reviewer to the appropriate section. Protective sheet covers are used on documents throughout the portfolio.	

(continued)

TABLE 14.1 Modifiable Scoring Rubric for a Portfolio Assignment (continued)

Category (Points Possible)	Does Not Meet Expectations	Nearly Meets Expectations	Meets Expectations	Exceeds Expectations	Comments
	E-portfolio: The main page is inaccessible or difficult to access. One or more of the required sections are missing or the reviewer is unable to access required sections. Many sections lack supportive documentation.	**E-portfolio:** The main page is easily accessed. All of the required sections are clearly identified and accessible. One or more of the sections are lacking any supportive documentation within the section.	**E-portfolio:** The main page is easily accessed. All required sections are clearly identified and accessible with minimal acceptable documentation included in each section.	**E-portfolio:** The main page is easily accessed. All required sections are clearly identified, accessible, and the pages are well developed with multiple sources of supportive documentation provided in each.	
	≤7	8	9	10	
Student information (10)	Significant student information required is missing such as student name, picture, and name of school or expected graduation date leading to difficulty identifying the student, or the student contact information is incomplete or missing, or personal interests are presented in an unprofessional manner.	Most of the student information required is present but does not include one or more the following: student name, picture, name of school, expected graduation date, or method for contacting the student. The missing information does not interfere with being able to clearly identify the student or personal interests are provided in an unprofessional manner.	All student information required is clear and complete, including student name, picture, name of school, and expected graduation date. A method for contacting the student is provided. A personal interest is provided in a professional manner.	All student information is clear and complete, including student name, professional picture, name of school, and expected graduation date. Several methods of contacting the student are provided. Personal interests are provided in a professional manner, which enhances the portfolio.	

	≤10	11–12	13–14	15
Resume/ curriculum vitae (CV) (15)	The student's CV is not provided or the student's CV has substantial unexplained gaps and misspellings. The content of the CV is disorganized and incomplete. The CV does not have a professional appearance.	The student's CV has minor gaps or misspellings. The CV contains information about education and work history, although the presentation of the information is disorganized. Overall, the CV lacks a professional appearance.	The student's CV is complete and organized at a basic level with education and work history included. Information is slightly inconsistent in presentation in that some is succinct and other information is a bit excessive and this detracts slightly from the overall professional appearance.	The student's CV is complete and organized with education, work history, and accomplishments clearly and succinctly presented. The CV has a professional appearance.

	≤7	8	9	10
Professional documents (10)	No cover letter is included or the cover letter is unprofessional in appearance, content, or writing or the student fails to identify an interest in a specific position. The student does not identify contact information or a professional reference.	The cover letter is casual without attention to business format. The student identifies an interest in a position and provides one means of being contacted. The student provides one professional reference.	The cover letter is clearly written in business format and identifies interest in a specific position. The student provides two means of being contacted. The student provides two professional references.	The cover letter is engaging and clearly written in business format, and the student succinctly identifies interest in a specific position and explains why. The student provides several means to be contacted. The student provides three or more professional references.

(continued)

TABLE 14.1 Modifiable Scoring Rubric for a Portfolio Assignment (*continued*)

Category (Points Possible)	Does Not Meet Expectations	Nearly Meets Expectations	Meets Expectations	Exceeds Expectations	Comments
	≤7	8	9	10	
Career path (10)	The student's career path is unclear and professional interests are vague or nonexisting. There are no supportive data for potential interests provided. The student Identifies one type of professional contact or one place for potential employment.	The student's career path and interests are generic, with limited supporting information about the general career path. Identifies one professional contact with contact information, or identifies one place for potential employment with contact information provided.	The student's career path and interests are outlined and the student provides supporting information regarding the career path and required preparation. The student provides one professional contact with contact information and one place for potential employment with contact information.	The student's career path and interests are identified and described with supporting information regarding the career path and required preparation. The student provides two or more professional contacts with contact information and two or more places for potential employment with contact information.	

	<14	15–16	17–18	19–20
Course syllabus and student work products with reflections (20)	Copies of less than half of the syllabi from courses taken to date are included or less than half of the work product(s) and evaluations are included or there is limited to no self-reflections on learning regarding the work products presented.	A copy of most syllabi from courses taken to date are included and followed by some required work product(s) with evaluation and self-reflection from the assignments or self-reflections from several work products are missing.	A copy of each syllabus from all courses taken to date is included and followed by the required work product(s) with evaluation and self-reflection from the assignments. Self-reflections minimally address what the student learned through the experience and future application.	A copy of each syllabus from all courses taken to date is included and followed by the required work product(s) with evaluation and self-reflection from the assignments. Self-reflections address in detail what the student learned through completing the assignment and how it will be applied in the future.

	≤7	8	9	10
Self-assessment (10)	Little to no self-assessment is evident. The student self-identifies a strength or a weakness. The competency list developed is incomplete. A plan for personal/professional development is lacking or underdeveloped.	The student identifies a strength and a weakness. Provides a list of competencies with minimal gaps. A plan for personal/professional development is briefly outlined with at least one strategy identified to address the weakness.	The student describes at least two strengths, two weaknesses, and provides a list of competencies. A plan for personal/professional development is outlined with at least several strategies identified to address each weakness and utilize strengths.	The student explores multiple strengths and weaknesses and provides a list and description of competencies. A detailed plan for personal/professional development is identified with multiple strategies identified to address weaknesses and utilize strengths.

(continued)

TABLE 14.1 Modifiable Scoring Rubric for a Portfolio Assignment (*continued*)

Category (Points Possible)	Does Not Meet Expectations	Nearly Meets Expectations	Meets Expectations	Exceeds Expectations	Comments
	≤7	8	9	10	
Professionalism and creativity (10)	There are multiple spelling and punctuation errors that impact readability. The font size and/or style are inconsistent and impair readability. Color contrasts appear random and detract from the portfolio continuity and professional appearance. The visuals support the written information less than half of the time.	There are several minor spelling/punctuation errors that do not impact readability. The font size and/or style are inconsistent throughout the portfolio. Color contrasts are used inconsistently and detract from continuity. The visuals support written information a majority of the time, but not all are professional in appearance.	There are minimal errors in spelling, word usage, or punctuation that do not impact readability. The font size and/or style are appropriate. There is a good use of color and contrast. The visuals support written information on most pages.	There are no errors in spelling, word usage, or punctuation. The font size and/or style are appropriate. There is a good use of color and contrast throughout. The visuals support and enhance the written information.	
Total points possible: 100	**Score and summary comments:**				

212

manager. If a hard copy of the portfolio is provided for evaluation, return the portfolio along with a hard copy of the completed rubric to the student.

CONCLUSION

A portfolio as a course or program assignment provides students a means to track their academic growth and development over time; highlight their skills, competencies, and accomplishments; self-reflect; organize professional documents; and plan for transitioning into a professional role. A portfolio as an assignment serves as a method for assessment and evaluation of the student's level of achievement of course learning objectives and/or program outcomes. Student portfolios also provide the educator the opportunity to assess and evaluate effectiveness and completeness of a course and/or curriculum.

REFERENCES

Abel, W. M., & Freeze, M. (2006). Evaluation of concept mapping in an associate degree nursing program. *Journal of Nursing Education, 45*(9), 356–364.

Adema-Hannes, R., & Parzen, M. (2005). Concept mapping: Does it promote meaningful learning in the clinical setting? *College Quarterly, 8*(3), 1–7.

All, A., & Havens, R. (1997). Cognitive/concept mapping: A teaching strategy for nursing. *Journal of Advanced Nursing, 25*(6), 1210–1219.

Allen, D., & Tanner, K. (2006). Rubrics: Tools for making learning goals and evaluation criteria explicit for both teachers and learners. *CBE Life Science Education, 5*(3), 197–203.

Anderson, I. (2009). Avoiding plagiarism in academic writing. *Nursing Standard, 23*(18), 35–37.

Baglione, S., & Nastanski, M. (2007). The superiority of online discussions: Faculty perceptions. *The Quarterly Review of Distance Education, 8*(2), 139–150.

Bastable, S. B. (2014). *Nurse as educator: Principles of teaching and learning for nursing practice* (4th ed.). Burlington, MA: Jones & Bartlett Learning.

Bean, J. C., & Peterson, D. (1998). Grading classroom participation. *New Directions for Teaching and Learning, 74*, 33–40.

Beitz, J. M. (1998). Concept mapping. Navigating the learning process. *Nurse Educator, 23*(5), 35–41.

Bender, T. (2012). *Discussion-based online teaching to enhance student learning: Theory, practice, and assessment* (2nd ed.). Sterling, VA: Stylus.

Bickes, J. T., & Schim, S. M. (2010). Righting writing: Strategies for improving nursing student papers. *International Journal of Nursing Education Scholarship, 7,* 1–10.

Billings, D. M., & Halstead, J. (2011). *Teaching in nursing: A guide for faculty* (4th ed.). Philadelphia, PA: Saunders/Elsevier.

Bischof, J. (2013). APNs taking the next step: Disseminating practice information via effective poster presentations. *The Nurse Practitioner, 38*(2), 1–4.

Bloom, B. S., Englehart, M. B., Furst, E. J., Hill, W. H., & Krathwohl, D. R. (1956). *Taxonomy of educational objectives: The classification of educational goals. Handbook I: Cognitive domain.* New York, NY: Longmans Green.

Bolin, A. U., Khramtsova, I., & Saamio, D. (2005). Using student journals to stimulate authentic learning: Balancing Bloom's cognitive and affective domains. *Teaching of Psychology, 32*(3), 154–159.

Bramer, S. E. V., & Basting, L. D. (2013). Using a progressive paper to develop students' writing skills. *Journal of Chemical Education, 90*(6), 745–750.

Brookfield, S. (1987). *Developing critical thinkers. Challenging adults to explore alternative ways of thinking and acting.* San Francisco, CA: Jossey-Bass.

Byrne, M., Schroeter, K., Carter, S., & Mower, J. (2009). The professional portfolio: An evidence-based assessment method. *The Journal of Continuing Education in Nursing, 40*(12), 545–562.

Christenbery, T. L., & Latham, T. G. (2013). Creating effective scholarly posters: A guide for DNP students. *Journal of the American Association of Nurse Practitioners, 25,* 16–23.

Cizek, G. J. (2009). Reliability and validity of information about student achievement: Comparing large-scale and classroom testing contexts. *Theory into Practice, 48,* 63–71.

Clayton, L. H. (2006). Concept mapping: An effective, active teaching-learning method. *Nursing Education Perspectives, 27*(4), 197–203.

Critz, C. M., & Knight, D. (2013). Using the flipped classroom in graduate nursing education. *Nurse Educator, 38*(5), 210–213.

Croxall, B. (2010). *How to grade students' class participation.* Retrieved from http://chronicle.com/blogs/profhacker/how-to-grade-students-class-participation/23726

Daley, B., Shaw, C., Balistrieri, T., Glasenapp, K., & Piacentine, L. (1999). Concept maps: A strategy to teach and evaluate critical thinking. *Journal of Nursing Education, 38*, 42–47.

Dallimore, E. J., Hertenstein, J. H., & Platt, M. B. (2004). Classroom participation and discussion effectiveness: Student-generated strategies. *Communication Education, 53*(1), 103–115.

Davis, B. G. (1993). *Tools for teaching*. San Francisco, CA: Jossey-Bass.

deYoung, S. (2008). *Teaching strategies for nurse educators* (2nd ed.). Upper Saddle River, NJ: Prentice Hall.

Fallahi, C. R., Wood, R. M., Austad, C. S., & Fallahi, H. (2006). A program for improving undergraduate psychology students' basic writing skills. *Teaching of Psychology, 33*(3), 171–175.

Friedrich, D. B., Goncalves, A. M., Sa, T. S., Duque, D. R., & Oliveira, G. M. (2010). The portfolio as an evaluation tool: An analysis of its use in an undergraduate nursing program. *Revista Latino-Americana de Enfermagem, 18*(6), 1123–1120.

FriWassef, M. E., Riza, L., Maciag, T., Worden, C., & Belaney, A. (2012). Implementing a competency-based electronic portfolio in a graduate nursing program. *Computers in Nursing, 30*(5), 242–248.

Gerdeman, J. L., Lux, K., & Jacko, J. (2013). Using concept mapping to build clinical judgment skills. *Nurse Education in Practice, 13*(1), 11–17.

Gibbs, G. (1988). *Learning by doing: A guide to teaching and teaching methods*. Oxford: Further Education Unit, Oxford Brookes University.

Gilboy, N., & Kane, D. (2004). Unfolding case based scenarios: A method of teaching and testing the critical thinking skills of newly licensed nurses. *Journal of Emergency Nursing, 30*(1), 83–85.

Gothler, A. M. (2000). Developing written assignments. In L. J. Scheetz (Ed.), *Nursing faculty secrets* (pp. 155–159). Philadelphia, PA: Hanley & Belfus.

Green, K. H., & Emerson, A. (2007). A new framework for grading. *Assessment & Evaluation in Higher Education, 32*(4), 495–511.

Griffin, M. T. Q., & Novotny, J. M. (2012). *A nuts-and-bolts approach to teaching nursing* (4th ed.). New York, NY: Springer Publishing Company.

Grossman, S., Krom, Z. R., & O'Connor, R. (2010). Innovative solutions: Using case studies to generate increased nurse's clinical decision-making ability in critical care. *Dimensions of Critical Care Nursing, 29*(3), 138–142.

Gul, R. B., & Boman, J. A. (2006). Concept mapping: A strategy for teaching and evaluation in nursing education. *Nurse Education in Practice, 6*(4), 199–206.

Harrison, E. (2012). How to develop well-written case studies: The essential elements. *Nurse Educator, 37*(2), 67–70.

Harrison, P., & Fopma-Loy, J. (2010). Reflective journal prompts: A vehicle for stimulating emotional competence in nursing. *Journal of Nursing Education, 49*(11), 844–852.

Harrow, A. (1972). *A taxonomy of the psychomotor domain: A guide for developing behavioral objectives.* New York, NY: David McKay.

Hawks, S. J. (2012). The use of electronic portfolios in nurse anesthesia education and practice. *AANA Journal, 80*(2), 89–93.

Head, K. S., & Johnson, J. H. (2012). Evaluation of the personal development portfolio in higher education: An explorative study. *Nurse Education Today, 32,* 857–861.

Hill, C. (2006). Integrating clinical experiences into the concept mapping process. *Nurse Educator, 31,* 36–39.

Hobson, E. H. (1998, Summer). Designing and grading written assignments. *New Directions for Teaching and Learning, 1998* (74), 51–57.

Holliday, W. (2013). *How to create a concept map.* Retrieved from http://library.usu.edu/instruct/tutorials/cm/CMinstruction2.htm

Hong, L. P., & Chew, L. (2008). Reflective practice from the perspectives of the bachelor of nursing students in international medical university. *International Nursing Journal, 35*(3), 5–15.

Hubert, J. (2010). Collaborative learning and self-assessment through reflective writing. *International Journal of Nursing, 17*(5), 385–398.

Iwaoka, W. T., & Crosetti, L. M. (2007). Using academic journals to help students learn subject matter content, develop and practice critical reasoning skills, and reflect on personal values in food science and nutrition classes. *Journal of Food Science Education, 7,* 19–29.

Keeley, M. (1997). *Questioning and using cognitive structures.* Retrieved from http://faculty.bucks.edu/specpop/question.htm

King, M., & Shell, R. (2002). Teaching and evaluating critical thinking with concept maps. *Nurse Educator, 27*(5), 214–216.

Kostovich, C. T., Poradzisz, M., Wood, K., & O'Brien, K. L. (2007). Learning style preference and student aptitude for concept maps. *Journal of Nursing Education, 46*(5), 225–231.

Krathwohl, D. R. (2002). Revision of Bloom's taxonomy: An overview. *Theory into Practice, 41*(4), 212–264.

Krathwohl, D. R., Bloom, B. S., & Masia, B. B. (1964). *Taxonomy of educational objectives: The classification of educational objectives. Handbook II: The affective domain.* New York, NY: David McKay.

Kraus, S., & Sears, S. (2008). Teaching for the millennial generation: Student and teacher perceptions of community building and individual pedagogical techniques. *The Journal of Effective Teaching, 8*(2), 32–39.

Lane, J. (2007). *Case writing guide.* Retrieved from www.schreyerinstitute.psu.edu

Langley, M. E., & Brown, S. (2010). Perceptions of the use of reflective learning journals in online graduate nursing education. *Nursing Education Perspectives, 31*(1), 12–17.

LaRocco, S. A. (2010). Assisting nursing students to develop empathy using a writing assignment. *Nursing Educator, 35*(1), 10–11.

Li-Ling, H. (2004). Developing concept maps from problem-based learning scenario discussions. *Journal of Advanced Nursing, 48*(5), 510–518.

Linnell, K. M. (2010). Using dialogue journals to focus on form. *Journal of Adult Education, 39*(1), 23–28.

Loo, R. (2004). Kolb's learning styles and learning preferences: Is there a linkage? *Educational Psychology, 24,* 99–108.

Luckowski, A. (2003). Concept mapping as a critical thinking tool for nurse educators. *Journal for Nurses in Staff Development, 19*(5), 228–233.

Lunney, M., & Sammarco, A. (2009). Scoring rubric for grading students' participation in online discussions. *Computers, Informatics, Nursing, 27*(1), 26–31.

Martinson, D. L. (2009). Adjusting grades? Let ethics be your guide. *Kappa Delta Pi Record, 45*(3), 122–125.

Maznevski, M. L. (1996). *Grading class participation.* Retrieved from http://trc.virginia.edu/resources/grading-class-participation-2

McColgan, K., & Blackwood, B. (2009). A systematic review protocol on the use of teaching portfolios for educators in further and higher education. *Journal of Advanced Nursing, 65*(12), 2500–2507.

McDonald, M. E. (2014). *The nurse educator's guide to assessing learning outcomes* (3rd ed.). Burlington, MA: Jones & Bartlett Learning.

McMullan, M., Endacott, R., Gray, M. A., Jasper, M., Miller, C. M. L., Scholes, J., & Webb, C. (2003). Portfolios and assessment of competence: A review of the literature. *Journal of Advanced Nursing, 41*(3), 283–294.

Melvin, K. B. (1988). Rating class participation: The prof/peer method. *Teaching of Psychology, 15*(3), 137–139.

Moellenberg, K. K., & Aldridge, M. (2010). Sliding away from PowerPoint: The interactive lecture. *Nurse Educator, 35*(6), 268–272.

Moule, P., Judd, M., & Girot, E. (1998). The poster presentation: What value to the teaching and assessment of research in pre- and post-registration nursing course? *Nurse Education Today, 18*, 237–242.

Moyer, B. A., & Wittman-Price, R. A. (2008). *Nursing education: Foundations for practice excellence*. Philadelphia, PA: F. A. Davis.

Mueller, A., Johnston, M., & Bligh, D. (2002). Joining mind mapping and care planning to enhance student critical thinking and achieve holistic nursing care. *Nursing Diagnosis, 13*(1), 24–27.

Multhaup, K. S. (2008). *Peer and self-evaluation of participation in discussion*. Retrieved from http://uwf.edu/cutla/class_participation.cfm

National Association of Colleges and Employers. (2013). *The skills and qualities employers want in their class of 2013 recruits*. Retrieved from http://www.naceweb.org/s10242012/skills-abilities-qualities-new-hires.aspx?terms=job%20candidate%20skills

National Center for Case Study Teaching in Science. (2013). *Case types and teaching methods: A classification scheme*. Retrieved from http://sciencecases.lib.buffalo.edu/cs/collection/method.asp

National Council of State Boards of Nursing. (2013). *2013 NCLEX-RN detailed test plan – Educator version*. Retrieved from https://www.ncsbn.org/4235.htm?iframe=true&width=515&height

Nesbit, J. C., & Adesope, O. (2006). Learning with concept and knowledge maps: A meta-analysis. *Review of Educational Research, 76*, 413–448.

Nilson, L. B. (2010). *Teaching at its best* (3rd ed.). San Francisco, CA: Jossey-Bass.

Nitko, A. J., & Brookhart, S. M. (2011). *Educational assessment of students* (6th ed.). Boston, MA: Allyn & Bacon.

Novak, J. D., & Canas, A. J. (2008). *The theory underlying concept maps and how to construct them.* Retrieved from http://cmap.ihmc.us/publications/researchpapers/theorycmaps/theoryunderlying-conceptmaps.htm

Oermann, M., & Gaberson, K. (2014). *Evaluation and testing in nursing education* (4th ed.). New York, NY: Springer Publishing Company.

Oermann, M. H. (2002). Developing a professional portfolio in nursing. *Orthopaedic Nursing, 21*(2), 73–77.

Oermann, M. H. (2013). *Teaching in nursing and role of the educator.* New York, NY: Springer Publishing Company.

Oermann, M. H., Yarbrough, S. S., Saewert, K. J., Ard, N., & Charasika, M. (2009). Clinical evaluation and grading practices in schools of nursing. *Nursing Education Perspectives, 50*(4), 352–358.

O'Neill, G., & Jennings, D. (2012). *The use of posters for assessment: A guide for staff.* Retrieved from www.ucd.ie/t4cms/UCDTLA0039.pdf

Painter, D. (2011). *Assigning and assessing student presentations.* Retrieved from http://polkfacultycentral.com/student-presentations/assessing-and-grading

Parikh, S. B., Janson, C., & Singleton, T. (2012). Video journaling as a method of reflective practice. *Counselor Education and Supervision, 51,* 33–49.

Pope, G., Kleeman, J., McNamara, B., & Phaup, J. (2007). *The legal defensibility of assessments: What you need to know.* Retrieved from http://www.www.cedma-europe.org/newsletter%20articles/misc/Legal%20defensibility%20of%20assessments%20-%20What%20you%20need%20to%20know%20(Oct%202007).pdf

Popil, I. (2011). Promotion of critical thinking by using case studies as teaching method. *Nurse Education Today, 31,* 204–207.

Quinn H. J., Mintzes J. L., & Laws, R. A. (2004). Successive concept-mapping. *Journal of College Science Teaching, 33*(3), 12–16.

Roberts, S. T., & Goss, G. (2009). Use of an online writing tutorial to improve writing skills in nursing courses. *Nurse Educator, 34*(6), 262–265.

Rossetti, J., Oldenburg, N., Robertson, J. F., Coyer, S. M., Koren, M. E., Peters, B., . . . Musker, K. (2012). Creating a culture of evidence in nursing education using student portfolios. *International Journal of Nursing Education Scholarship, 9*(1), 1–14.

Rotenberg, R. (2012). *The art & craft of college teaching: A guide for new professors and graduate students* (2nd ed.). Walnut Creek, CA: Left Coast Press.

Schmidt, N. A., & Brown, J. M. (2012). *Evidence-based practice for nurses.* Sudbury, MA: Jones & Bartlett Learning.

Shatzer, M., Wolf, G. A., Hravnak, M., Haugh, A., Kikutu, J., & Hoffmann, R. L. (2010). A curriculum designed to decrease barriers related to scholarly writing by staff nurses. *The Journal of Nursing Administration, 40*(9), 392–398.

Siegrist, B., Garrett-Wright, D., & Abel, C. H. (2011). Poster presentations as a teaching strategy in web-based courses. *Nursing Education Perspectives, 32*, 198–199.

Smith, L. J. (2008). Grading written projects: What approaches do students find most helpful? *Journal of Education for Business, 83*(6), 325–330.

Sprang, S. M. (2010). Making the case: Using case studies for staff development. *Journal of Nursing Staff Development, 26*(2), E6–E10.

Strunk, W., & White, E. B. (2000). *Elements of style* (4th ed.). Needham Heights, MA: Longman.

Summers, K. (2005). Student assessment using poster presentations. *Paediatric Nursing, 17*(8), 24–26.

Svinicki, M., & McKeachie, W. J. (2011). *McKeachie's teaching tips: Strategies, research, and theory for college and university teachers* (13th ed.). Belmont, CA: Wadsworth Cengage Learning.

Task Oriented Question Construction Wheel Based on Bloom's Taxonomy. (2004). St. Edward's University Center for Teaching Excellence.

Taylor, L. A., & Littleton-Kearney, M. (2011). Concept mapping: A distinctive educational approach to foster critical thinking. *Nurse Educator, 36*(2), 84–88.

The Learning Management Corporation. (n.d.). *Developing clear learning outcomes and objectives.* Retrieved from http://www .thelearningmanager.com/pubdownloads/developing_clear_ learning_outcomes_and_objectives.pdf

The Teaching Center at Washington University in Saint Louis. (2009). *Increasing student participation.* Retrieved from http://teaching-center.wustl.edu/strategies/Pages/increasing-participation.aspx

Toofany, S. (2008). Critical thinking among nurses. *Nursing Management – UK, 14*(9), 28–31.

University of Maryland School of Nursing. (2013). *BSN program outcomes*. Retrieved from http://www.nursing.umaryland.edu/academic-programs/undergrad

University of Oregon. (2013). *Bloom's taxonomy of cognitive levels*. Retrieved from http://tep.uoregon.edu/resources/assessment/multiplechoicequestions/blooms.html

Vacek, J. E. (2009). Using a conceptual approach with a concept map of psychosis as an exemplar to promote critical thinking. *Journal of Nursing Education, 48*(1), 49–53.

Walker, L. O., & Avant, K. C. (1995). *Strategies for theory construction in nursing*. East Norwalk, CT: Appleton & Lange.

Walvoord, B. E., & Anderson, V. J. (1998). *Effective grading: A tool for learning and assessment*. San Francisco, CA: Jossey-Bass.

Weimer, M. (2011). *How much should class participation count toward the final grade?* Retrieved from http://www.facultyfocus.com/articles/teaching-professor-blog/how-much-should-class-participation-count-toward-the-final-grade

Weimer, M. (2012). *Student presentations: Do they benefit those who listen?* Retrieved from http://www.facultyfocus.com/articles/teaching-and-learning/student-presentations-do-they-benefit-those-who-listen

Wharrad, H. J., Allcock, N., & Meal, A. G. (1995). The use of posters in the teaching of biological sciences of an undergraduate nursing course. *Nurse Education Today, 15*, 370–374.

Wheeler, L. A., & Collins, S. K. (2003). The influence of concept mapping on critical thinking in baccalaureate nursing students. *Journal of Professional Nursing, 19*(6), 339–346.

Wilgis, M., & McConnell, J. (2008). Concept mapping: An educational strategy to improve graduate nurses' critical thinking skills during a hospital orientation program. *Journal of Continuing Education in Nursing, 39*(3), 119–126.